Current Cataract Surgical Techniques

Edited by Xiaogang Wang

Published in London, United Kingdom

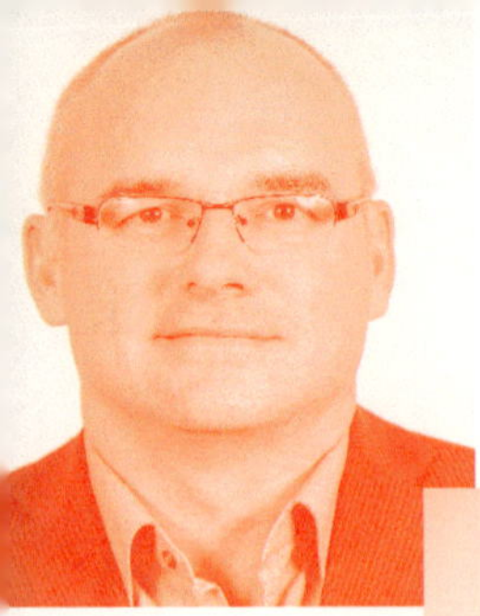
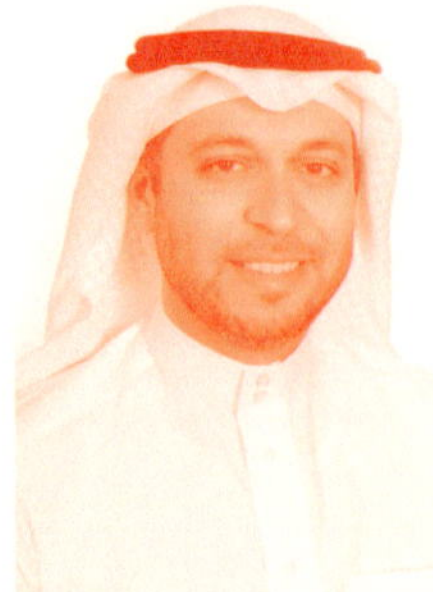
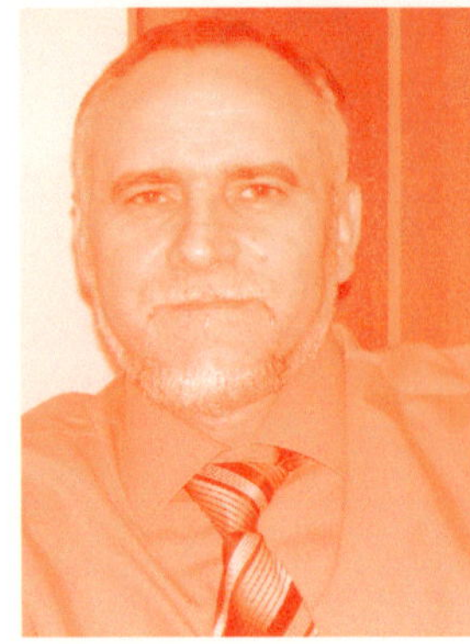
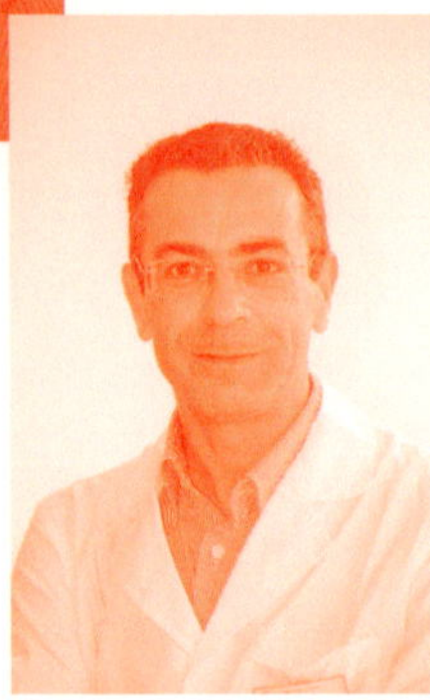
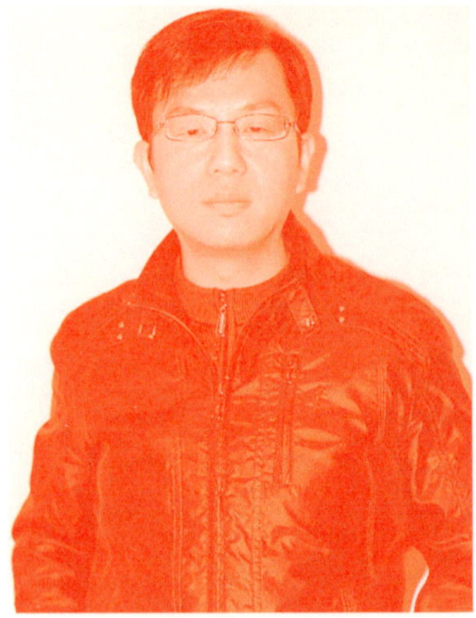
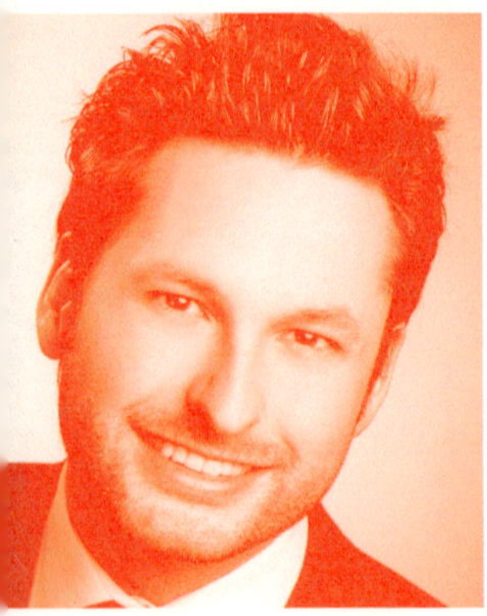
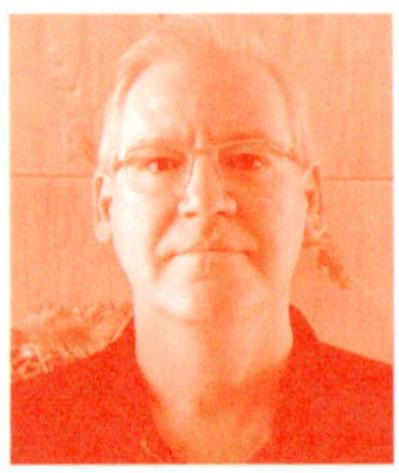

IntechOpen

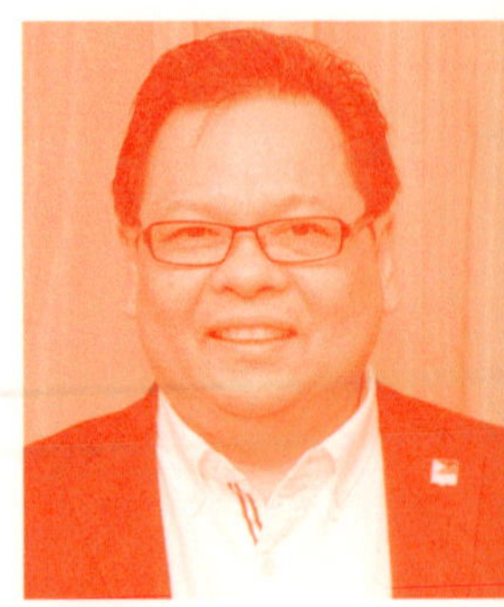
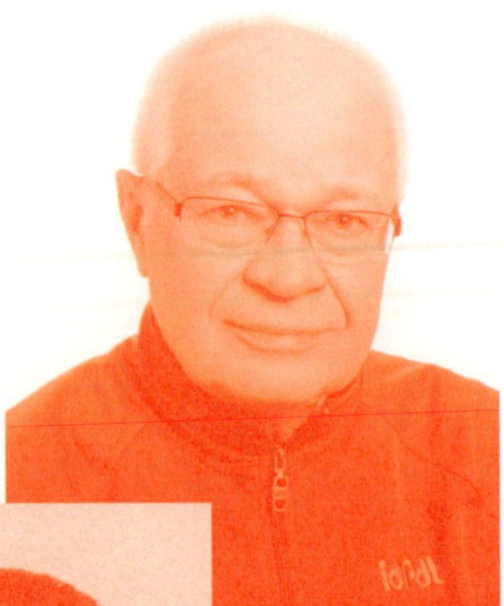
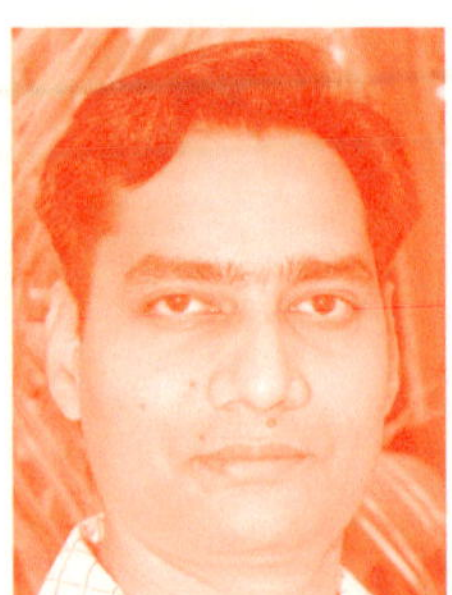
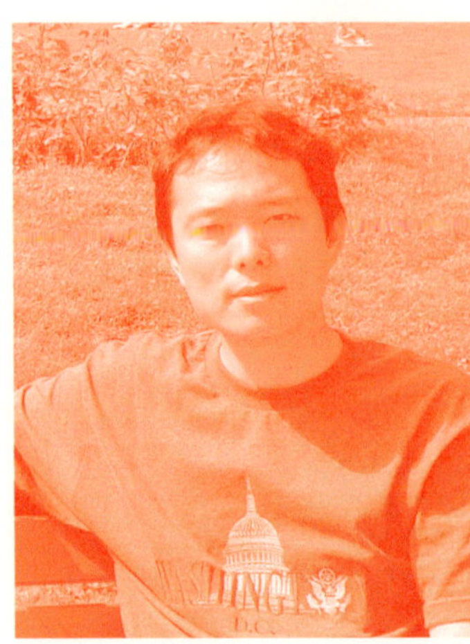
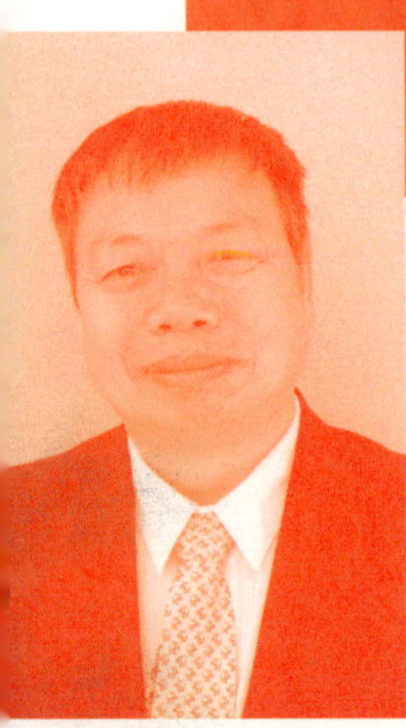
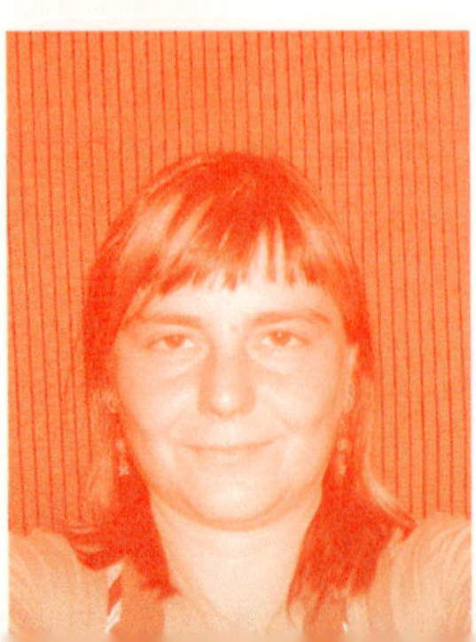

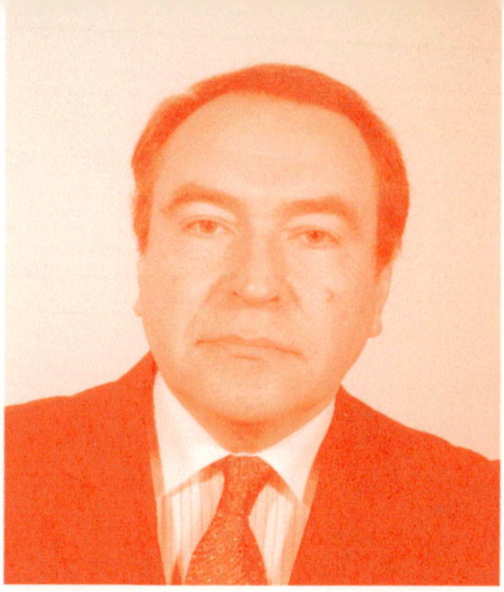

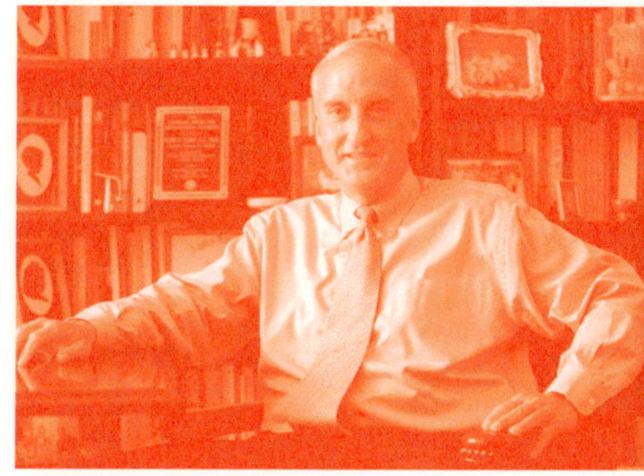

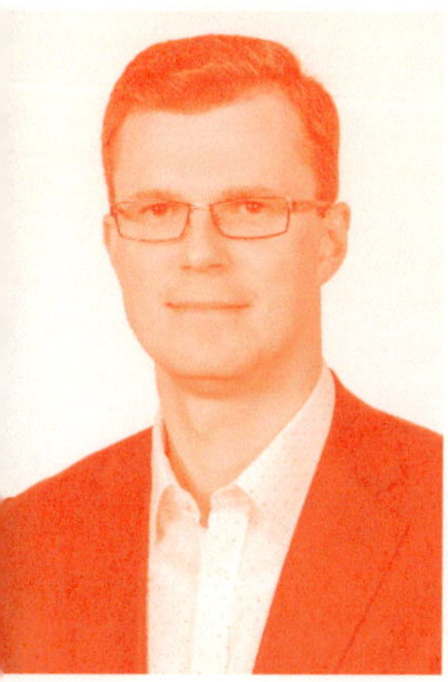

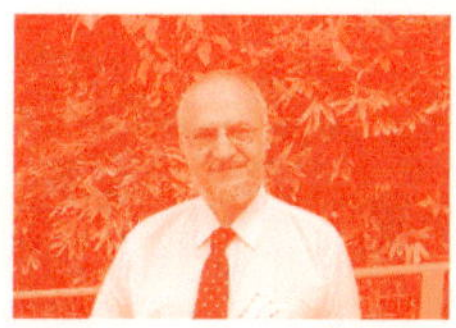

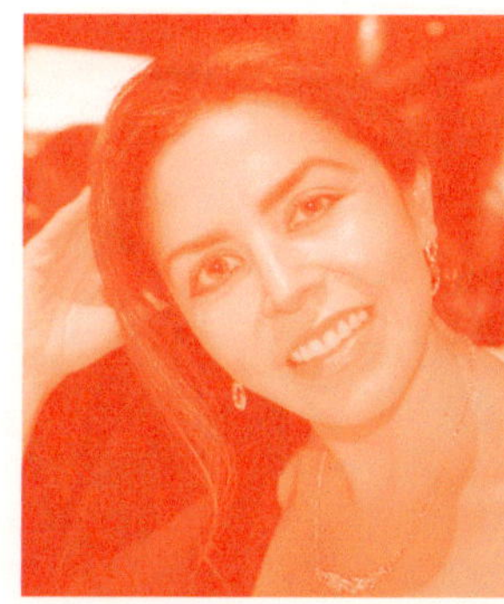

Supporting open minds since 2005

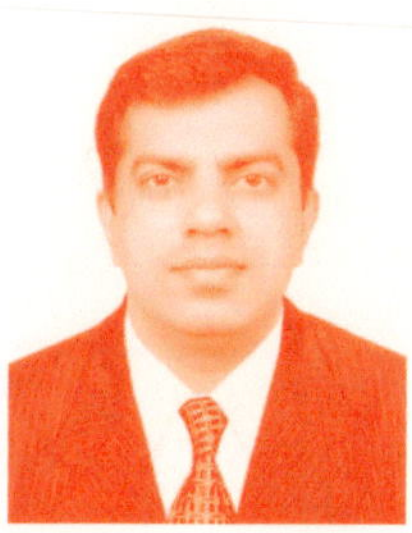

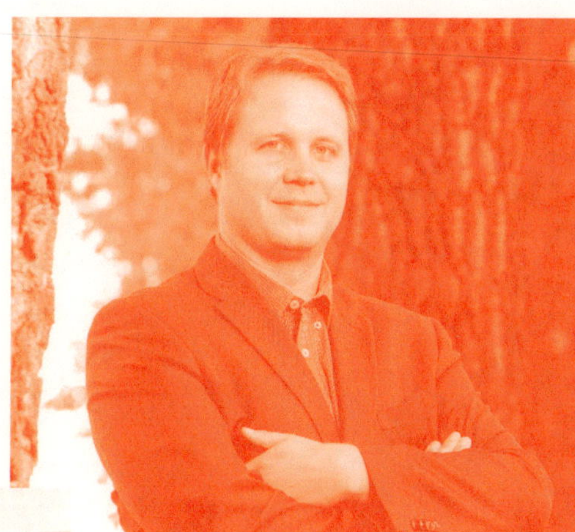

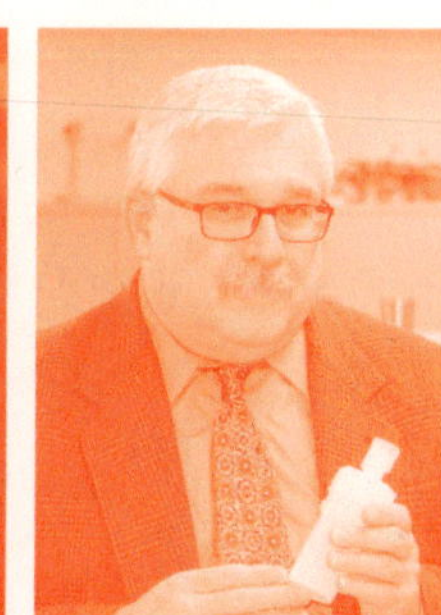

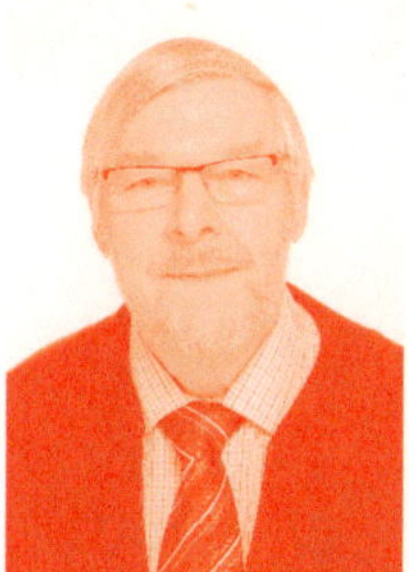

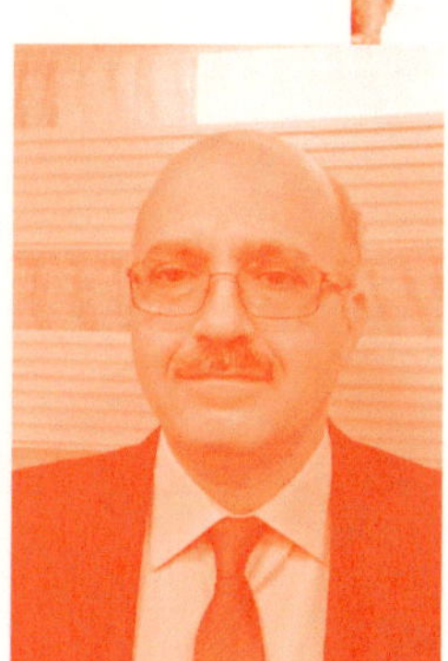

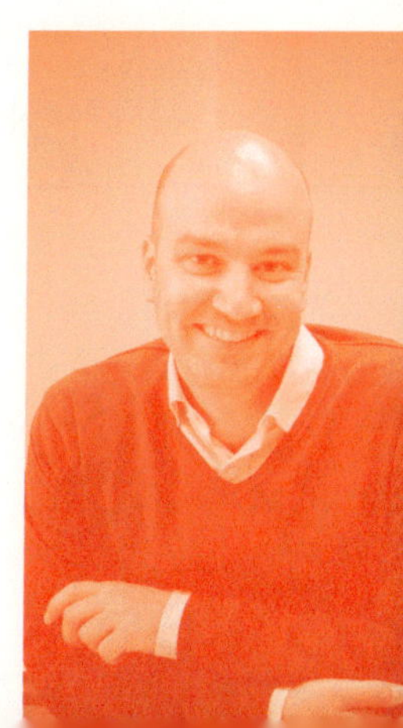

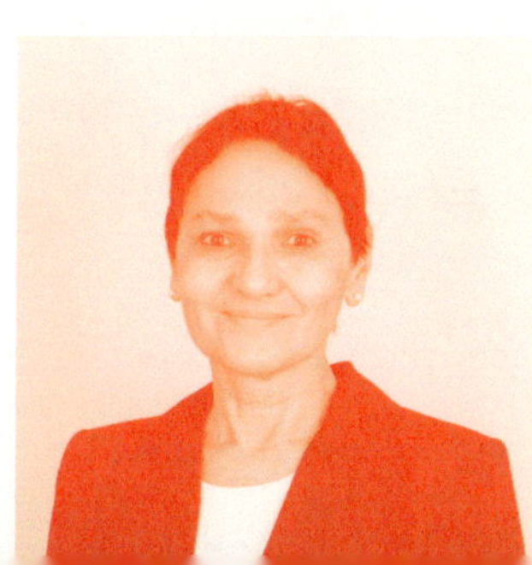

Current Cataract Surgical Techniques
http://dx.doi.org/10.5772/intechopen.92901
Edited by Xiaogang Wang

Contributors
Olivia Esteban Floria, Javier Mateo, Javier Lara Medina, Paula Casas, Francisco J. Ascaso, Humberto Dória Silva, Rostan Silvestre, Eduardo Dória Silva, Maria Tamires Dória Silva, Cristiana Pereira Dória, Cristiane Pereira Dória, Marina Aguilar Gonzalez, Jorge Vila Arteaga, Jose Marí Cotino, Georgios Labiris, Eirini-Kanella Panagiotopoulou, Liu Qian, Chen Xu, Minghui Deng, Song Chen, Xiaogang Wang

First published in London, United Kingdom, 2021 by IntechOpen
IntechOpen is the global imprint of INTECHOPEN LIMITED, registered in England and Wales, registration number: 11086078, 5 Princes Gate Court, London, SW7 2QJ, United Kingdom
Printed in Croatia

British Library Cataloguing-in-Publication Data
A catalogue record for this book is available from the British Library

Additional hard and PDF copies can be obtained from orders@intechopen.com

Current Cataract Surgical Techniques
Edited by Xiaogang Wang
p. cm.
Print ISBN 978-1-83968-674-0
Online ISBN 978-1-83968-675-7
eBook (PDF) ISBN 978-1-83968-676-4

For EU product safety concerns:
IN TECH d.o.o., Prolaz Marije Krucifikse Kozulić 3, 51000 Rijeka, Croatia, info@intechopen.com or visit our website at intechopen.com.

Meet the editor

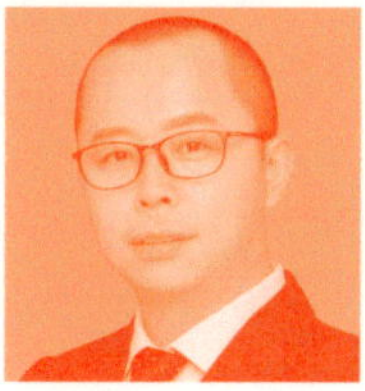

Dr. Xiaogang Wang, a faculty member of Shanxi Eye Hospital specializing in the treatment of cataract and retinal disease and a tutor for postgraduate students of Shanxi Medical University, worked in the COOL Lab as an international visiting scholar under the supervision of Dr. David Huang and Yali Jia from October 2012 through November 2013. Dr. Wang earned an MD from Shanxi Medical University and a Ph.D. from Shanghai Jiao Tong University. Dr. Wang was awarded two research project grants focused on multimodal optical coherence tomography imaging and deep learning in cataract and retinal disease, from the National Natural Science Foundation of China. He has published around 30 peer-reviewed journal papers and four book chapters and co-edited one book.

Contents

Preface

Phacoemulsification cataract surgery is one of the most frequently performed surgical procedures in the world. With advances in surgical techniques, the era of refractive cataract surgery has arrived. However, the surgeon should still focus on basic skills such as central continuous curvilinear capsulorhexis (CCC), phaco-chop techniques, and others. Moreover, specific challenging cases related to surgical techniques and surgical plan design, such as combining cataract surgery with microinvasive glaucoma surgery, cataract surgery in post-vitrectomized eyes, visual impairment caused by monovision surgical design, premium intraocular lens (IOL) implantation in cases of posterior capsule rupture and previous corneal refractive surgery, and capsular shrinkage syndrome of retinitis pigmentosa, should also be considered. The book also discusses issues of selecting candidates for IOL and pseudophakic presbyopia correction.

This book is fortunate to have outstanding contributors from different countries. We believe that the content of *Current Cataract Surgical Techniques* has a practical and clinical interest in clinical ophthalmology. Moreover, we hope that this book provides a timely answer to some current clinical needs.

Xiaogang Wang
Shanxi Eye Hospital,
Taiyuan, China

Section 1

Basic Skills

Chapter 1

Continuous Curvilinear Capsulorhexis

Liu Qian

Abstract

Continuous curvilinear capsulorhexis (CCC) is an important step in of modern phacoemulsification, which has crucial influence on the surgical process and prognosis. In this chapter, we mainly discuss following aspects: Preoperative preparation, Effects of incision on capsulorhexis, Capsulorhexis, Special cases of capsulorhexis and Capsulorhexis assisted by femtosecond laser. The problem need to pay attention and the solution way in above aspects will be elaborated.

Keywords: continuous, circular, centered, capsulorhexis, cataract

1. Introduction

Thomas Neuhann and Howard Gimbel, considered as pioneers in the development of the centered continuous curvilinear capsulorhexis (CCC) technique, first published their paper on the technique in 1990 [1]. The use of CCC technique makes the rim of the anterior capsule (AC) much stronger and decreases the risk of tearing, thus providing a solid foundation for applying the "chip and flip," "divide and conquer," "phaco chop," and "phaco pre-chop" techniques. What is more, the IOL could be more correctly positioned and stability with the centered continuous curvilinear anterior opening [2–5]. In terms of improving the prognosis, CCC technique could supply a continuous opening with more smooth edges [6]. The morphology of anterior capsule affect position of lens and refractive outcome greatly [7]. CCC helps maintain the intraocular lens (IOL) in the correct position and overlaped by anterior capsule as showed in **Figure 1** which providing a more predictable effective lens position (ELP) [6]. In addition, The CCC technique could reduce the incidence of posterior capsular opacification (PCO) [8–10]. With the current widespread-use of multi-focus intraocular lenses and astigmatism-correcting intraocular lenses, Cataract surgery has entered the refractive age. Centered CCC(CCCC) play a crucial role in obtaining good postoperative visual quality. Tilt and decentration of the IOL can decrease visual acuity which could result in astigmatism [11, 12]. Okada et al. [13] confirmed that decentration of optic center by 0.4 mm could produce 0.25D change in spherical equivalent.

In this chapter, we will elaborate on several aspects include: preoperative preparation; the effects of incision on capsulorhexis. The two parts above mainly discuss the tools, head position of patient, exposure of surgical field of vision, red reflex of microscope, hand position of surgeon and importance of incision. Then capsulorhexis technique and special cases of capsulorhexis will be interpreted. In the end, we will introduce the advantage of femtosecond laser system in capsulorhexis and precautions.

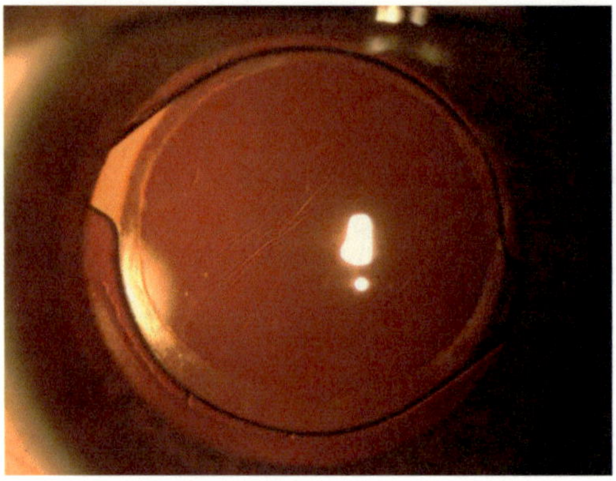

Figure 1.
Color photo of patient 3 months after CCCC. The margin of optic region was overlaped by anterior capsule full-circlely.

2. Preoperative preparation

2.1 Tools for CCC

Initially, a type of irrigating cystotome (designed by Charles Kelman) and a needle were employed in CCC. The first forceps, specifically used to conduct capsulorhexis, were designed by Peter Utrata in 1988,and are still used today.

Forceps were designed in different lengths, with columnar and flat handle (**Figure 2**) and the tips were curved and flat (**Figure 3**). Compared with columnar handle, the flat handle is easier for thumb and index finger to hold and middle finger to support and relatively more lighter. After the viscoelastic agent was injected into the front chamber, the anterior capsule is flattened. The flat tip has more room to move around in the anterior chamber. The curved tip generate height difference in the anterior chamber. Limited by the incision, the movement of curved tip is restricted. The choice of length, depends on the habit and hand size of the operator and the last choice of columnar and flat handle or curved and flat tip depends on the habit too.

Aim to reduce the incidence of infection after operation especially to decrease surgically induced astigmatism and the influence on corneal optical performance in refractive cataract surgery, corneal incision size was reduced from over 3 mm to less

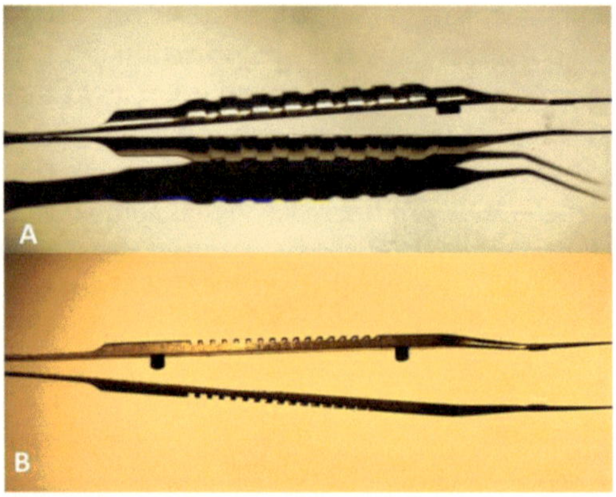

Figure 2.
Different designs of forceps handle. A is columnar and B is flat.

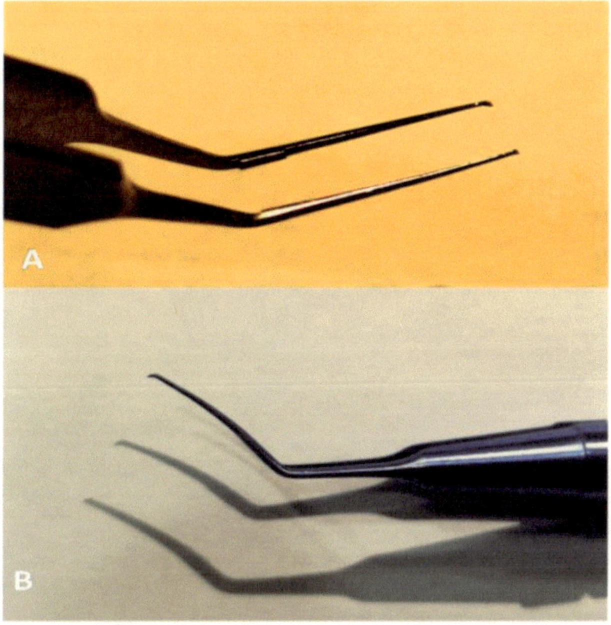

Figure 3.
Different designs of forceps tip. A is flat and B is curved.

than 2 mm [14–19]. The related equipment is also required to be further improved. Smaller incisions limit the movement of traditional capsular forceps. Calladine-Inamura Capsulorhexis Forceps increases the opening and closing range of the tip in the anterior chamber by the hinge design on the forearm as showed in **Figure 4** to complete capsulorhexis through small incision. Ikeda MICS Capsulorhexis Forceps is tube designed with small diameter as 0.7 mm (showed in **Figure 5**) could enter anterior chamber for capsulorhexis through small paracentesis.

Scales of 5 mm and 2.5 mm are marked on some of the flat-tipped forceps, as shown in **Figure 6**, which can be useful as a measurement reference for the operator.

2.2 Patient's head position

The position of the head is vital to ensure the centrality of the AC opening. The patient's head should be kept horizontal for the lens plane to remain horizontal

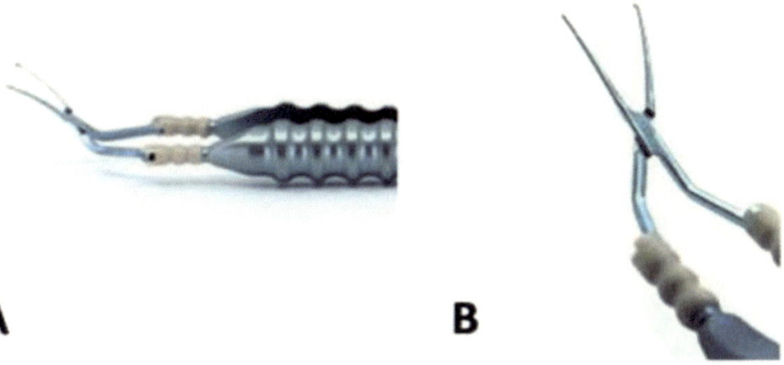

Figure 4.
Calladine-Inamura Capsulorhexis forceps. Hinge design on the forearm in a and the detail in B.

(**Figure 7**). The AC opening could be decentered downwards if the jaw is too elevated (**Figure 8**), or upwards if the forehead is too elevated (**Figure 9**).

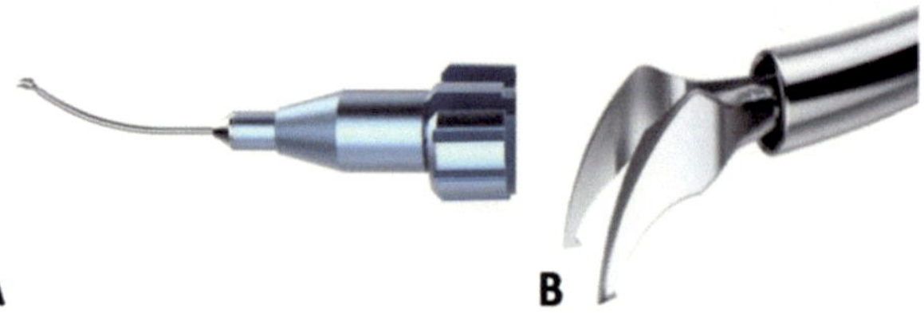

Figure 5.
Ikeda MICS Capsulorhexis forceps. Tube design without joint in A and the detail of tip in B.

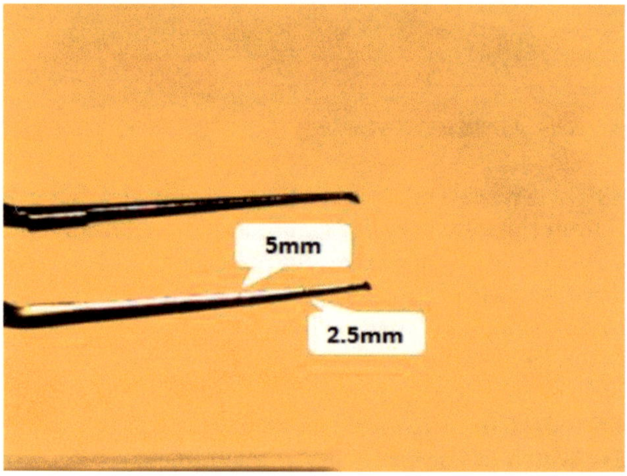

Figure 6.
The scaleis marked on the tip of forceps as scratches. The distal one is 2.5 mm, the proximal is 5 mm.

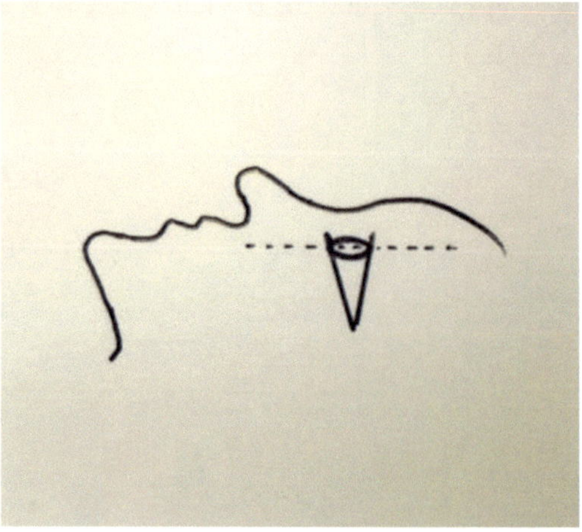

Figure 7.
The plane of the lens should be kept level by adjusting the position of head before operation.

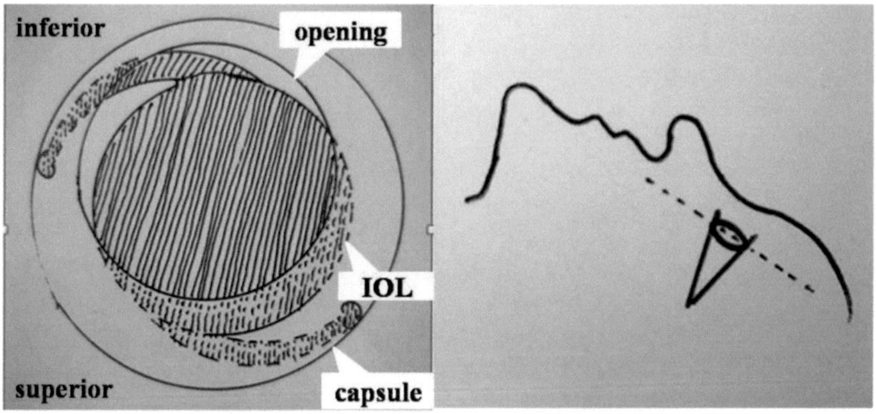

Figure 8.
The AC opening would be decentered towards inferior if the jaw is too elevated.

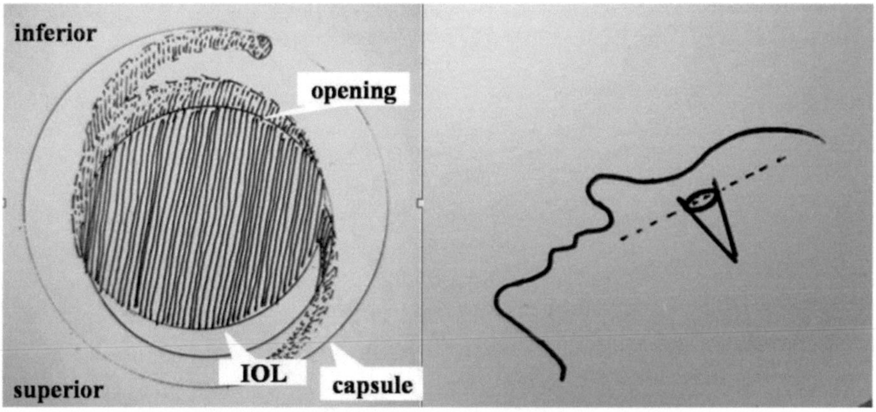

Figure 9.
The AC opening would be decentered towards superior if the forehead is too elevated.

2.3 Surgical field of vision

The pupils must be fully dilated to expose the surgical field. One drop of 0.5%tropicamide is instilled every 15 min (four times), to maintain the diameter of the pupil greater than 6.0 mm.

The rare cases in which cataracts are complicated with uveitis, the pupil cannot be dilated adequately because the iris is atrophic and inelastic. In such cases, the pupil can be stretched by two choppers, as shown in **Figure 10**, which is known as the pupil-stretch technique. Moreover, alternative devices and techniques are available. For example the iris can be fixed by iris hooks through a series of side-incisions to dilate the pupil (**Figure 11**), and the use of the Malyugin ring can reduce the number of side incisions required (**Figure 12**). There are also many other pupil expansion devices, such as Hydro view Iris Protector Ring, B-HEX Pupil Expander, I-Ring pupil expander etc., can be used in clinic.

However, the use of instruments or pupil-stretch technique can lead to tears of the iris muscle fiber, resulting in pupil malformation and even the risk of hemorrhage as show in **Figure 10** (red arrow). In such cases, coreoplasty can be performed using Vannas capsulotomy scissors, as shown in **Figure 13**.

Moreover, when the pupillary area of chronic uveitis is adhered to the AC by an exudative membrane, capsulorhexis forceps could be used to dilacerate the

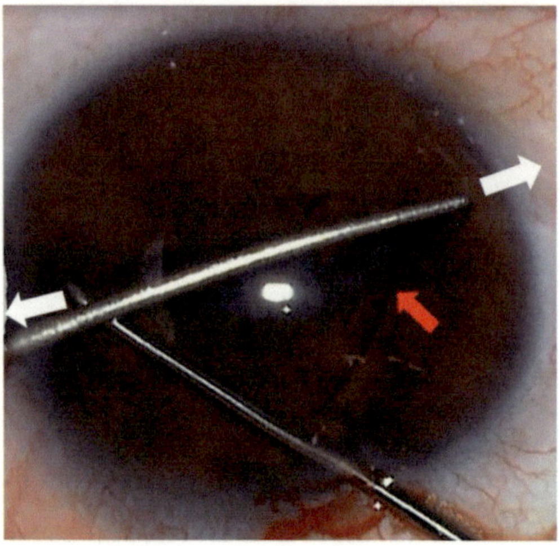

Figure 10.
To stretch the pupil in the opposite direction (white arrow) with two chopping hook. The relevant side-effect are hemorrhage (red arrow) and tansformation of pupil after operation.

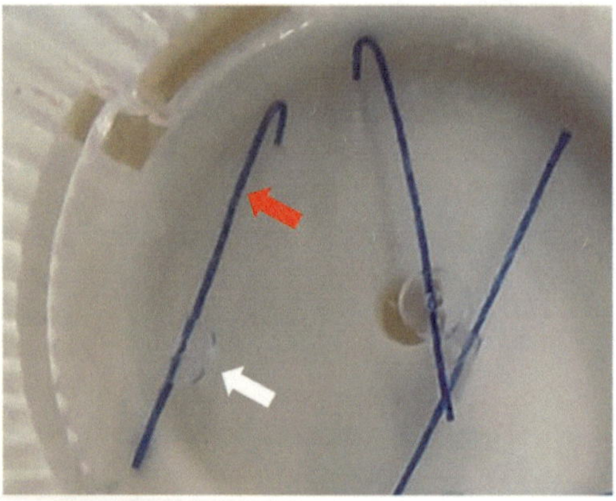

Figure 11.
Iris hooks to fix the iris through side incision which is composed of a hook (red arrow) and gasket (white arrow).

membrane (**Figure 14**). After both these procedures, the pupils can be dilated injection of a viscoelastic agent.

2.4 Red reflex during surgery

The red reflex test, which is performed using a microscope, is very important at each step of cataract surgery. It allows the surgeon to clearly see the capsulorhexis path by illuminating the AC (white arrow in **Figure 15**), and visualization of the path can be enhanced by adjusting the ratio of coaxial to paraxial light on the microscope (**Figure 16**).

In cases of mature or hyper mature cataracts, the light reflects off the posterior segment, generating a retro-illumination of the AC, which is insufficient for correctly performing capsulorhexis. In such cases, Trypan blue dye could be used to stain the AC.

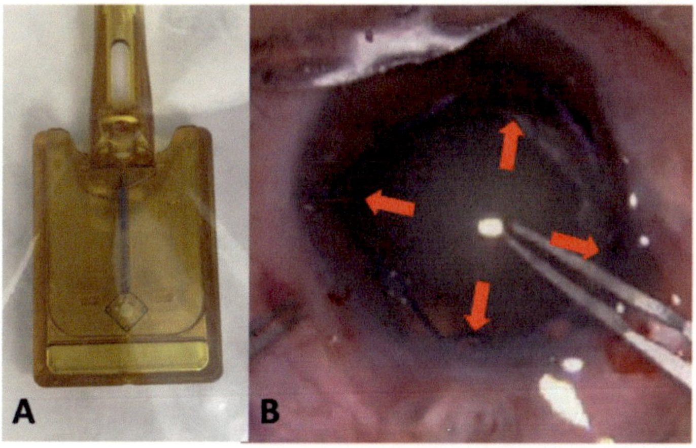

Figure 12.
Malyugin ring after disinfection and sealing is showed in A. Malyugin ring stretch the pupil during operation as showed in B (red arrow).

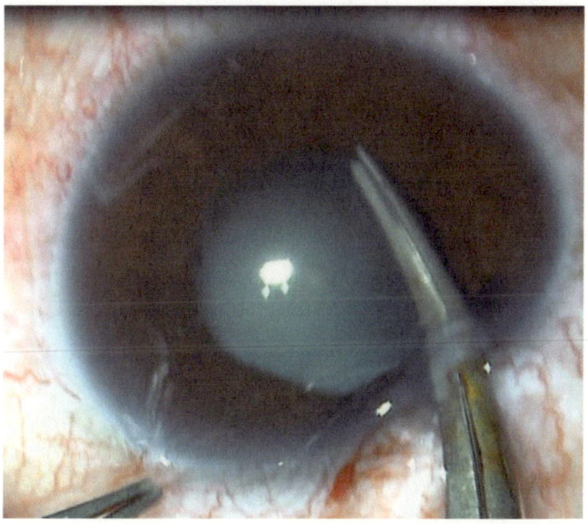

Figure 13.
Coreoplastyis applied by capsulotomy Vannas scissors to amplify the vision field.

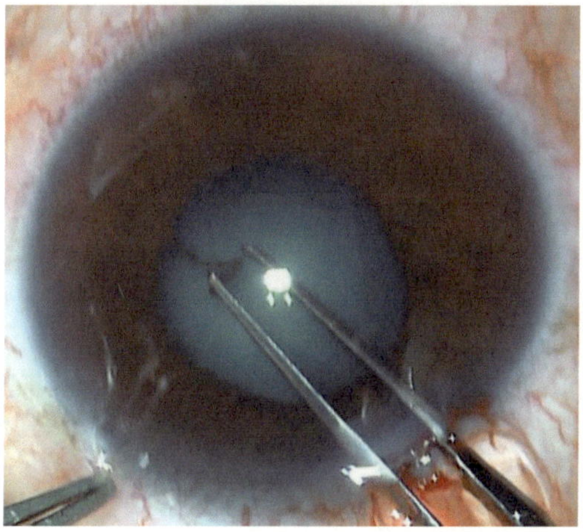

Figure 14.
Capsulorhexis forceps is used to tear the membranes to remove its restriction on the pupil.

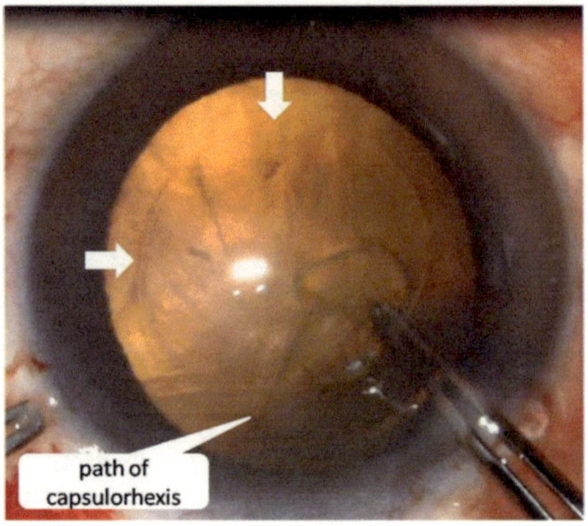

Figure 15.
Capsulorhexis path is clear with good red reflex (white arrow).

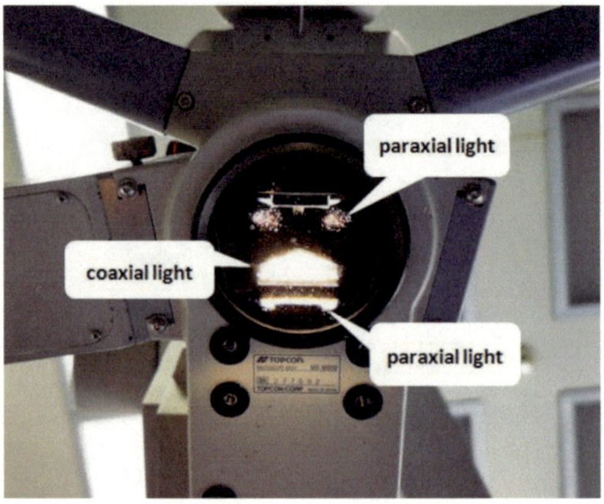

Figure 16.
Coaxial light and paraxial lights on the operation microscope.

2.5 Hand position

To avoid wrist dangling, the surgeon's hands or wrists should rest steadily against the patient's forehead. This will allow the surgeon's hands to move synchronously with the patient's head if the they move head abruptly. The angle at which the hands placed varies according to the practitioner's habits.

3. Effects of incision on capsulorhexis

An ideal surgical incision is the fundamental prerequisite for successful capsulorhexis. In Europe and America, a temporal incision is preferred, while in Asia it is mostly performed at an 11 o' clock position. Regardless of the orientation, when the incision is made, the direction of the tunnel knife should be along the meridian of the cornea, as shown in **Figure 17**.

A meridional incision does not limit the movement of capsular forceps, which ensures that the anterior opening is centered and perfectly round. When the incision deviates from the meridian, the boundaries of the inner incision will limit the track for the capsulorhexis forceps as shown in **Figure 18**.

In addition, if the incision is too close to the center of the cornea, the range will be affected, leading to a small and off-center capsulorhexis, as shown by the red arrows in **Figure 19**.

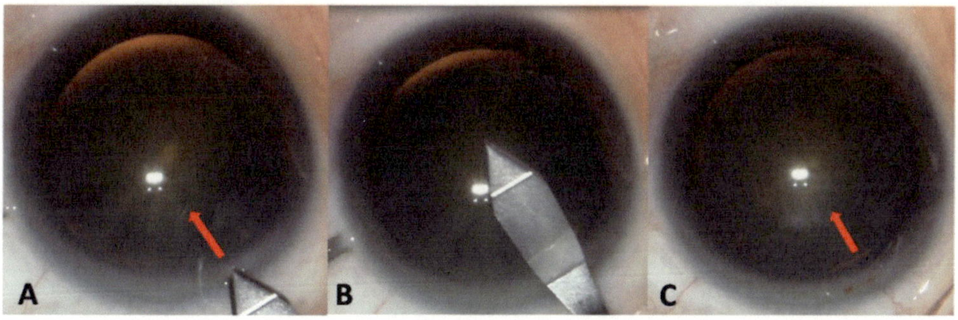

Figure 17.
The direction of incision should along meridian direction (C) from positioning (A) to the process of making the incision (B).

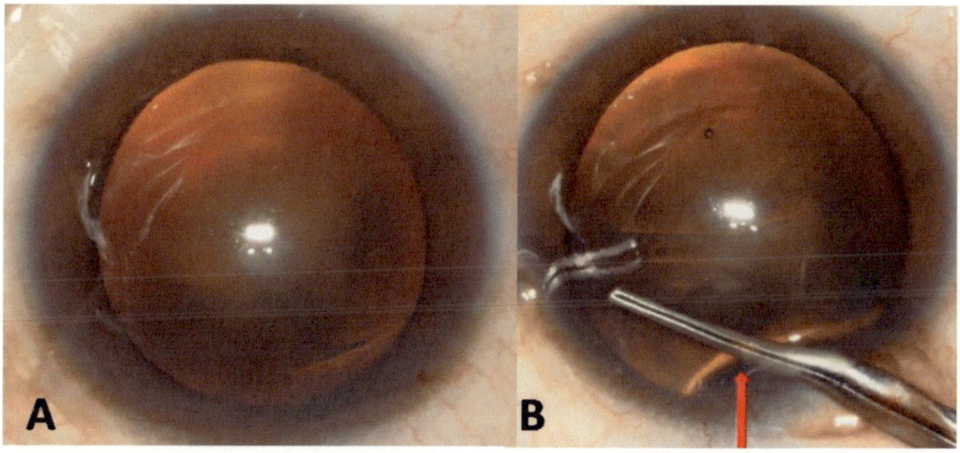

Figure 18.
Incision deviates from the meridian showed in A. the boundaries of deflective inner incision limit the movement of capsulorhexis forceps as showed in B.

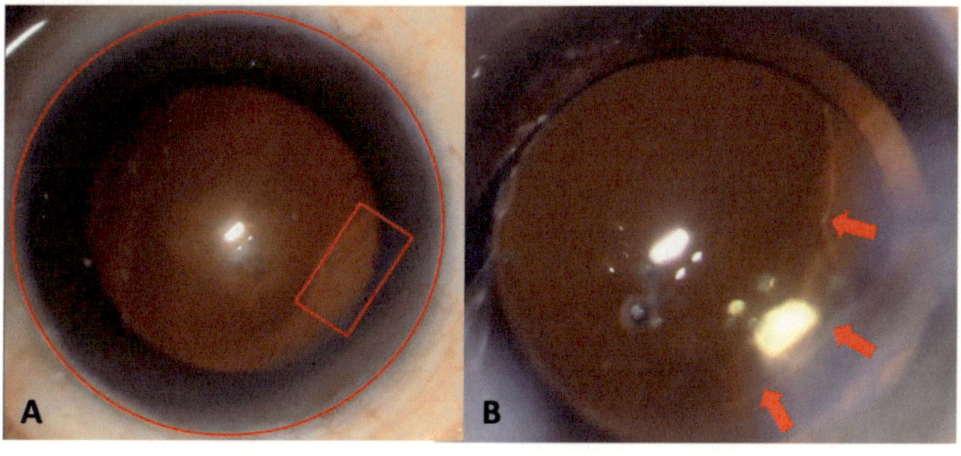

Figure 19.
Incision (red box) is too close to the center of the cornea relative to the limbus (red circle). The irregular AC opening (red arrow) followed the non-ideal incision.

4. Capsulorhexis

4.1 Viscoelastic injection

When a viscoelastic agent is injected into the eye, the needle should move inside out, while filling the whole anterior chamber with the viscoelastic to flatten the AC. Otherwise, the path of the capsulorhexis would slide in the direction of the suspensory ligament.

4.2 Bimanual coordination

Coordinate your hands, hold the tweezers in your dominant hand and slightly fixate the eyeball to maintain the cornea in the middle. The hand holding the tweezers should be soft and not put pressure on the eyes. Otherwise, the viscoelastic agent can extrude from the incision, resulting in uneven force on the AC and capsular tear. However, too much pressure on the eyeball will cause folds on the cornea, which affects the surgical field of vision.

4.3 The production of the lamella

The process of capsulorhexis is equivalent to drawing a circle. With the eye in position, consider the focal point reflected by the microscope light as the center, and tear the forceps from this point (red circle in **Figure 20**) to open the AC, with an outward radius of approximately 2.5 mm.

4.4 Capsulorhexis technique

The limbus can be used as reference to guide the capsulorhexis [20]. For the unexperienced surgeon, the technique is difficult given the narrow diameter of 5–5.5 mm. To aid the process, the marks on forceps in **Figure 6** or the marks made on the cornea before initiation of capsulorhexis, can be used for guidance.

The following points should be considered during capsulorhexis:

a. If excessive pressure is applied by the forceps on the internal incision, the viscoelastic agent could spill out from the incision site. This would leave the

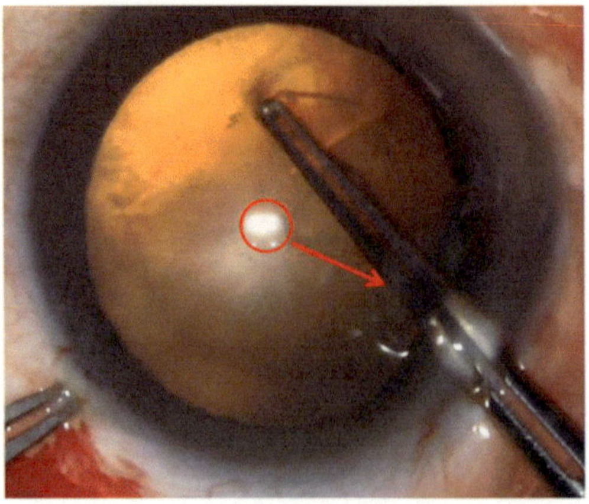

Figure 20.
The light spot (red cirlce) would be center of capsule if the position of head and eye maintain level. The radius of capsulorhexis is showed as red arrow.

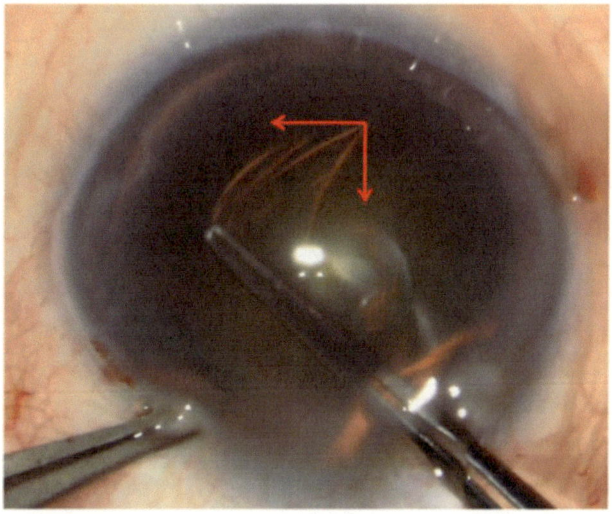

Figure 21.
The force of capsulorhexis is composed of forces in two direction as showed by red arrows. One is along the tangent of the circle, and the other is towards the center of the circle.

anterior chamber partially filled, and the resulting unbalanced forces applied on the AC, will cause capsulorhexis failure.

b. The trajectory of the capsulorhexis will depend on the balance of two forces exerted during the movement of the forceps by the surgeon, as shown in **Figure 21** by red arrows. One is the tearing force along the tangent of the circle, and the other is the pulling force perpendicular to the tangent, towards the center of the circle. Only when the two forces are balanced, will the trajectory be correct and the capsulorhexis completed successfully. If the tearing force along the tangent of the circle is larger, the trajectory of the capsulorhexis would shift laterally, causing a tear. If the pulling force is larger, the trajectory of capsulorhexis would deviate towards the center, resulting in a very small capsulorhexis.

c. A skilled surgeon can complete the capsulotomy in 3 to 4 attempts, while a beginner should increase the number of attempts and stop before the capsule trajectory cannot be controlled. Extra care should be taken at the joint, and an additional capsulotomy may be added if necessary.

d. During the movement, avoid lifting the forceps too high, to avoid scratching the corneal endothelium.

5. Special cases of capsulorhexis

5.1 Capsulorhexis in children

Congenital cataracts in children can be a challenge for surgeons, and should not be attempted by beginners, for several reasons:

a. The AC of children is more flexible, which makes it difficult to cut with forceps. The discission needle made by 1 ml syringe is the preferred instrument in this case, as shown in **Figure 22**.

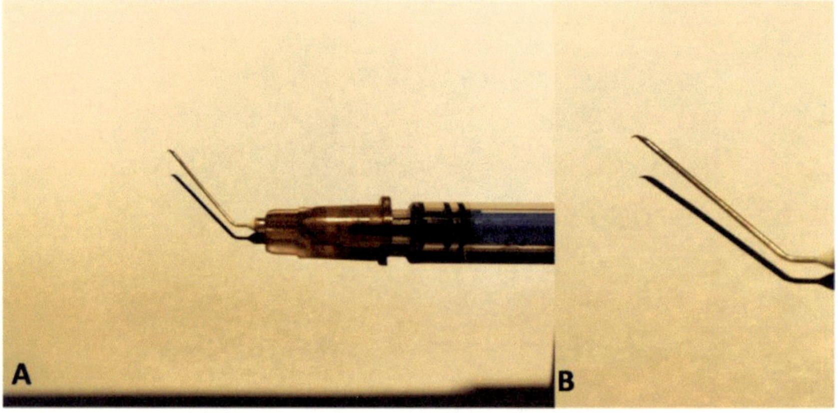

Figure 22.
A showed the discission needle made by 1 ml syringe. B showed the detail of the needle.

b. Owing to the increased toughness and flexibility of the AC, the trajectory of capsulorhexis can be difficult to control. The pulling force should be slightly increased to avoid tearing and an oversized opening.

c. Cataracts with congenital lens abnormality are usually associated with suspensory ligament anomaly, which can be a challenge even for a skilled operator.

5.2 Uveitis complicated cataract

The challenge in this situation is the difficulty of pupil dilation due to iris degeneration caused by uveitis, which has a significant impact on the surgical field of vision. The measures recommended for this situation have been already mentioned in the **surgical field of vision** section.

5.3 Mature cataract

In mature cataracts, the capsular membrane is relatively brittle and often accompanied by intumescent lens, as shown in **Figure 23**.

Due to the excessive expansion of the surface, the AC often tears-out, forming the Argentinian flag sign. To avoid this, the method of capsule decompression is recommended as follows:

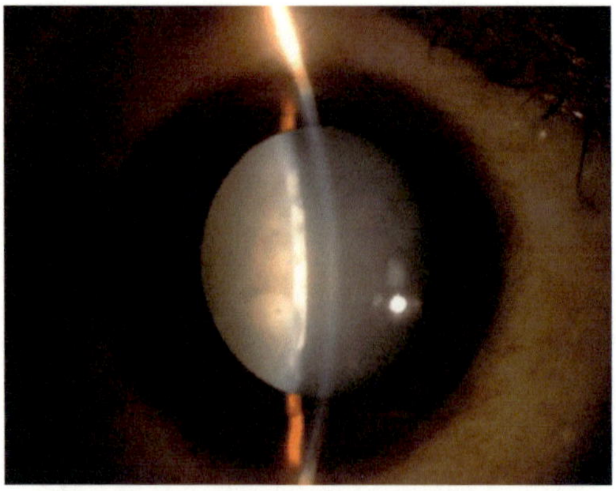

Figure 23.
Color photo of white cataract with intumescent lens and shallow anterior chamber.

a. Dye the capsule with Trypan blue to increase visibility

b. Puncture the central area of the AC with the tip of a needle or forceps as A in **Figure 24**, with a resulting liquefied cortical efflux (red arrow in B of **Figure 24**). A blunt needle can then be used to clear this efflux.

c. Alternatively a discission needle can be used to puncture the AC and then clear the liquefied cortex under the AC directly. Remember to bevel the needle downwards and to maintain the operation in the central area of the AC as C in **Figure 24**.

d. When the liquefied cortex is cleared, the central area of the AC will collapse (D in **Figure 24**). At this point, the AC can be flattened by injection of viscoelastic, and capsulorhexis initiated. The process of capsulorhexis could be then divided into two steps as needed, beginning with a small opening, and the then extending the radius to approximately 2.5 mm.

5.4 The challenge of small pupil and flabby suspensory ligament

A disease that often causes difficulty with capsulorhexis is exfoliation syndrome, because of two clinical aspects. Firstly, the pupils cannot be dilated past 5 mm,

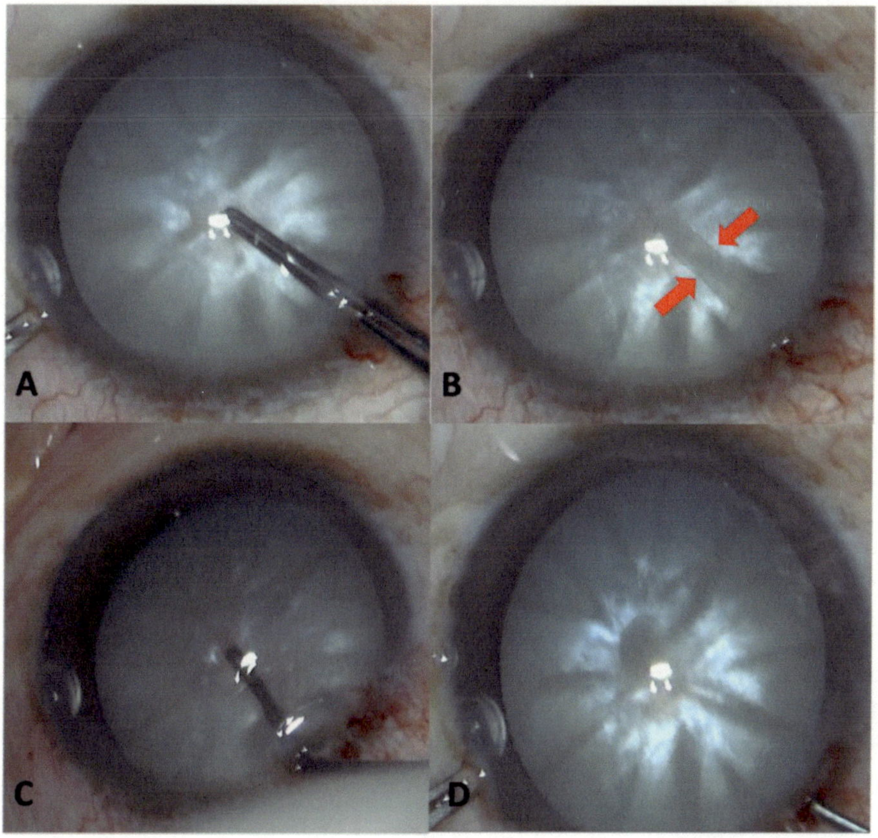

Figure 24.
Decompression of intumescen lens. To pierce the intumescent AC with the tip of capsulorhexis forceps (A). The liquefied cortex spills out (red arrows in B). Discission needle was applied to clear the liquefied cortex beneath AC (C). AC collapse appeared as larger annular reflections (D).

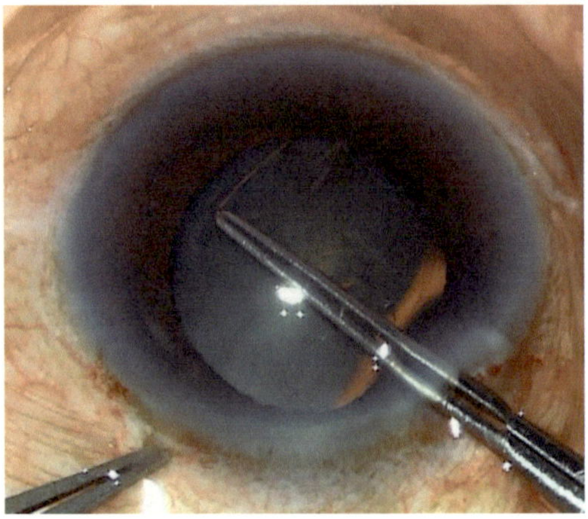

Figure 25.
The pupil is too small to expose the trajectory of the capsulorhexis. Skilled surgeons could perform a blind capsulorhexis.

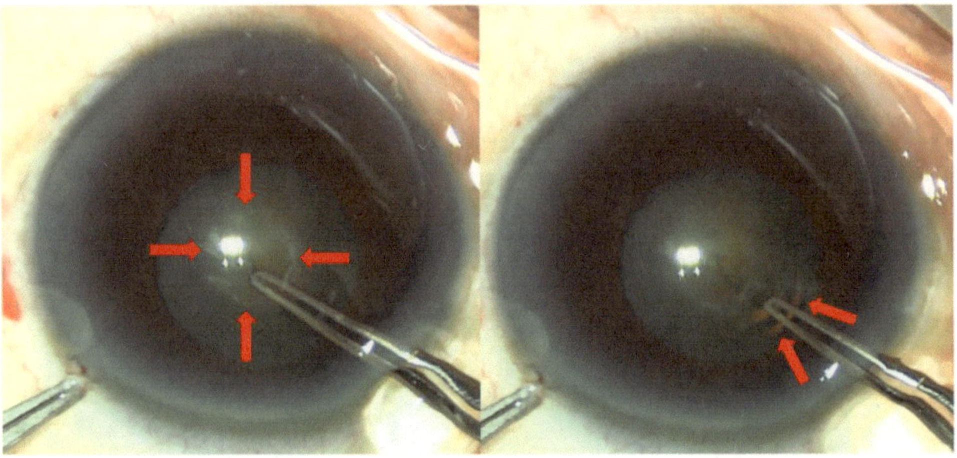

Figure 26.
Suspensory ligament of exfoliation syndrome is extremely flabby which could appear as the radial and wrinkled reflections during capsulorhexis (red arrow).

generating an insufficient red reflex for the operator to perform the procedure comfortably. The Malyugin ring, as mentioned in the section on the surgical field of vision, can be used in such situations. However, skilled surgeons often perform a blind capsulorhexis. The trajectory of the capsulorhexis is covered by the iris, as shown in **Figure 25**.

The other difficulty is extreme relaxation or even rupture of the suspensory ligament, which can be difficult to detect, even with UBM (Ultrasound Biomicroscopy). As the pupil cannot be dilated large enough and therefore the condition of suspensory ligaments around the capsule is not clear. However, the extent of the suspensory ligament relaxation can be judged by the folds caused by the tip of the capsular tweezers when touching the surface of the AC during capsulorhexis as showed in **Figure 26**.

When such a situation occurs, the surgeon should be careful, and the number of capsulorhexis should be appropriately increased to improve controllability. This method is also suitable for small pupils in diabetic patients and patients with prostatitis treated with Finasteride. Beginners should be aware of this disease and refer the cases to experienced surgeons.

6. Capsulorhexis assisted by femtosecond laser

Femtosecond laser capsulorhexisis superior in accuracy and precision compared with manual capsulorhexis, as well as the tensile strength of the capsule opening. An accurate circular, continuous and centered capsulorhexis as achieved by a femtosecond system cannot be achieved manually [21] (**Figure 27**). Because of these advantages, capsulorhexis assisted by a femtosecond laser is even more critical for premium IOLs. Presently, femtosecond laser surgery is also used in mature, traumatic, and for other cataract patients with suspensory ligament abnormalities [22–26].

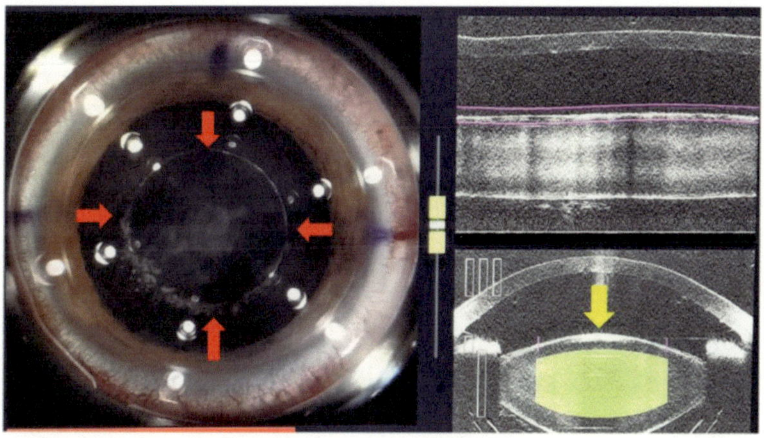

Figure 27.
The display interface of femtosecond laser during capsulorhexis. A perfect AC opening (red arrow) was conducted. Lens plane was also displayed by anterior OCT (yellow arrow).

This system greatly reduces the risk of capsulorhexis with due attention to the following recommendations:

1. The patient needs to be able to cooperate.

2. The patient's head and eye position should remain absolutely horizontal, as shown in **Figure 5**. Excessive upturn and downturn can lead to failure of capsulorhexis. Therefore, patients with head tremor and uncooperative eye position should be cautious. We can refer to the surface of the lens shown in anterior OCT of this system as yellow arrow in **Figure 27**.

3. The pupil must be dilated to at least 5 mm.

7. Conclusion

As cataract surgery enters the refractive age, the criteria "continuous, circular, and centered" have become the basic requirement of the capsulorhexis technique. Therefore, it is extremely important for the surgeon to master the technique of capsulorhexis.

Conflict of interest

The authors declare no conflict of interest.

Author details

Liu Qian
Department of Cataract, Shanxi Eye Hospital, Taiyuan, Shanxi, China

*Address all correspondence to: liuuqian@126.com

References

[1] Gimbel HV, Neuhann T. Development, advantages, and methods of the continuous circular capsulorhexis technique. J Cataract Refract Surg. 1990;16(1):31-7.

[2] Wyględowska-Promieńska D, Jaworski M, Kozieł K, Packard R. The evolution of the anterior capsulotomy. Videosurgery Miniinv. 2019;14(1):12-18.

[3] Gimbel HV, Neuhann T. Development, advantages, and methods of the continuous circular capsulorhexis technique. J Cataract Refract Surg. 1990; 16:31-7.

[4] Gimbel HV, Neuhann T. Continuous curvilinear capsulorhexis.J Cataract Refract Surg. 1991;17:110-1.

[5] T Neuhann. Theory and surgical technic of capsulorhexis. Klin Monbl Augenheilkd. 1987;190(6):542-5.

[6] Bhavana Sharma, Robin G Abell, Tarun Arora, Tom Antony, Rasik BVajpayee. Techniques of anterior capsulotomy in cataract surgery. Indian Journal of Ophthalmology. 2019;64(4):450-460.

[7] Kranitz K, Takacs A, Mihaltz K. Femtosecond laser capsulotomy and manual continuous curvilinear capsulorrhexis parameters and their effects on intraocular lens centration. J Refract Surg. 2011;27:558-63.

[8] HollickEJ, Spalton DJ, MeacockWR. The effect of capsulorrhexis size on posterior capsular opacification: One-year results of a randomized prospective trial. Am J Ophthalmol. 1999;128:271-9.

[9] Aykan U, Bilge AH, Karadayi K, Akin T. The effect of capsulorhexis size on development of posterior capsule opacification: Small (4.5 to 5.0 mm) versus large (6.0 to 7.0 mm). Eur J Ophthalmol. 2003;13:541-5.

[10] Ravalico G, Tognetto D, Palomba M. Capsulorhexis size and posterior capsule opacification. J Cataract Refract Surg. 1996;22:98-103.

[11] Hayashi K, Hayashi H. Effect of anterior capsule contraction on visual function after cataract surgery. J Cataract Refract Surg. 2007; 33(11):1936-1940.

[12] Wirtitsch MG, Findl O, Menapace R, Kriechbaum K, Koeppl C, Buehl W, et al. Effect of haptic design on change in axial lens position after cataract surgery. J Cataract Refract Surg. 2004;30:45-51.

[13] Okada M, Hersh D, Paul E, van der Straaten D. Effect of centration and circularity of manual capsulorrhexis on cataract surgery refractive outcomes. Ophthalmology. 2014;121:763-70.

[14] Chee SP, Bacsal K. Endophthalmitis after microincision cataract surgery. J Cataract Refract Surg. 2005;31:1834-5.

[15] Alió J, Rodríguez-Prats JL, Galal A, Ramzy M. Outcomes of microincision cataract surgery versus coaxial phacoemulsification. Ophthalmology. 2005;112:1997-2003.

[16] Elkady B, Piñero D, Alió JL. Corneal Incision Quality in Microincisional Cataract Surgery (MICS) vs. Microcoaxial Phacoemulsification. J Cataract Refract Surg. 2009;35:466-74.

[17] El Kady B, Alió J, Ortiz D, Montalbán R. Corneal aberrations after microincision cataract surgery. J Cataract Refract Surg. 2008;34:40-5.

[18] Yao K, Tang X, Ye P. Corneal astigmatism, high order aberrations, and optical quality after cataract surgery: Microincision versus small-incision. J Refract Surg. 2006;22:S1079-82.

[19] Jiang Y, Le Q, Yang J, Lu Y. Changes in corneal astigmatism and high order aberrations after clear corneal

tunnel phacoemulsification guided by corneal topography. J Refract Surg. 2006;22:S1083-8.

[20] Wang X, Dong J, Deng M. Limbus-centered marking technique-assisted continuous circularcapsulorhexis. Medicine (Baltimore). 2021 Jan 15;100(2):e24109.

[21] Friedman NJ, Palanker DV, Schuele G, Andersen D, Marcellino G, Seibel BS, Batlle J, Feliz R, Talamo JH, Blumenkranz MS, Culbertson WW. Femtosecond laser capsulotomy. J Cataract Refract Surg. 2011;37(7): 1189-1198.

[22] Pei-Wei Huang, Wei-Hsuan Huang, Yuan-Che Tai, Chi-Chin Sun. Femtosecond laser-assisted cataract surgery in a patient with traumatic cataract and corneal opacity after LASIK: a case report. BMC Ophthalmol. 2020;20(1):218.

[23] Soon-Phaik Chee, Melissa H Y Wong, Aliza Jap. Management of Severely Subluxated Cataracts Using Femtosecond Laser-Assisted Cataract Surgery. Am J Ophthalmol. 2017;173:7-15.

[24] Armando S. Crema, Aileen Walsh, Iris S. Yamane, Bruna V. Ventura, Marcony R. Santhiago. Femtosecond Laser-assisted Cataract Surgery in Patients With Marfan Syndrome and Subluxated Lens. J Refract Surg. 2015;31(5):338-341.

[25] Jeewan S Titiyal, Manpreet Kaur, Archita Singh, Tarun Arora, Namrata Sharma. Comparative evaluation of femtosecond laser-assisted cataract surgery and conventional phacoemulsification in white cataract. Clin Ophthalmol. 2016;22(10):1357-64.

[26] Danmin Cao, Yong Wang, Rong Lei, Mahmood Khan, Li Wang. Femtosecond laser-assisted cataract surgery in a spherophakic lens: An unusual case report. Medicine (Baltimore).2019;98 (44):e17426.

Section 2

Challenging Situations

Chapter 2

Cataract Surgery Combined with Trabecular MIGS (Minimally Invasive Glaucoma Surgery)

Marina Aguilar González, Jorge Vila Arteaga and Jose Marí Cotino

Abstract

Cataract surgery decreases significantly and with maintained effect intraocular pressure (IOP) in both normal eyes as in eyes with glaucoma. In patients with cataracts and glaucoma, it can be performed, isolated or in combination with other techniques, such as the following: minimally invasive glaucoma surgery (MIGS) in patients with mild/moderate glaucoma that do not require a high tensional decrease; and conventional glaucoma surgery techniques in patients with advanced glaucoma. Although lower than with conventional techniques, MIGS trabecular surgery has a good IOP lowering effect and provides some of the following advantages: a more physiological approach; little traumatic; without bleb; and it does not limit other techniques in the future. Different techniques that combinated or not with cataract surgery facilitate the exit of aqueous humor through the trabecular meshwork (TM) have been described. Our aim in this chapter is to review the newest of them, such as the following: iStent; ELT (Excimer Laser Trabeculostomy); kahook; ABiC; and OMNI.

Keywords: cataract surgery, glaucoma surgery, MIGS, iStent, ELT, Kahook, ABiC, OMNI

1. Introduction

It has been shown that after phacoemulsification in eyes with and without glaucoma, there is a decrease in IOP in relation to the preoperative one, with a decrease of up to 8.5 mmHg, 34% of the preoperative IOP, in eyes with glaucoma and IOP between 29 and 23 mmHg and 3.4 mmHg; and 18% of the IOP in eyes with preoperative IOP lower than 20 mmHg [1]. Moreover, the decrease in IOP is maintained up to 10 years follow-up without influence of the age of the patients [1]. Therefore, we can affirm that the cataract extraction, regardless of the surgical technique used, provides a reduction in preoperative IOP, maintained during follow-up, which is related to preoperative, both in normal eyes and in ocular hypertensive with or without treatment, and even in eyes with glaucoma and hypotensive medical treatment. Therefore, cataract surgery can be considered as an antiglaucomatous surgical technique, which could the indicated treatment in hyperopic eyes and adequate glaucoma control with medical treatment and in glaucomatous patients, with correct medical control, if we do not pursue a large decrease in IOP [2].

However, when a big IOP decrease is required or in the case of advanced glaucomas, we will use the classic surgical techniques for the treatment of glaucoma: trabeculectomy

IntechOpen

or nonpenetrating glaucoma surgery, as they present the highest hypotensive efficacy (but also a higher rate of complications than other less invasive techniques).

As an intermediate step, in mild or moderate glaucomas that do not require a high tensional decrease but in which an additional decrease in IOP than that obtained with isolated cataract surgery is needed, we can associate MIGS techniques with cataract surgery, since they offer good tensional responses (although smaller than those obtained with classical glaucoma surgeries) with a lower complication rate (both in number and severity) than with classical surgical techniques. All MIGS have in common a better postoperative recovery compared to other more invasive filtering procedures, the absence of complications associated with the bleb, the respect of the conjunctiva that will allow future techniques if required and the possibility of being performed easily in combination with cataract surgery.

In the following chapter, we are going to talk about the role of the trabecular approach and the MIGS techniques that use this approach associated with cataract surgery.

2. Anatomy of the trabecular meshwork

As we know, there are three ways of draining the aqueous humor [3]:

1. The conjunctival pathway.

2. The trabecular pathway.

3. The suprachoroidal pathway.

All three routes can be surgically approached both ab interno and ab externo.

The trabecular pathway is the physiological drainage pathway and it is where most of the keys of the pathophysiology of many types of glaucoma lie.

The trabecular pathway allows the aqueous humor to pass from the anterior chamber to the systemic circulation and we should see it like a dynamic mechanism instead of like a static mechanism.

1. The first structure in contact with the aqueous humor is the trabecular meshwork (TM). In the TM we differentiate three zones [3]:

    a. The uveal TM (**Figure 1**): it is located adjacent to the anterior chamber and is arranged in bands that extend from the root of the iris and the ciliary body to the peripheral cornea.

    b. The corneo-scleral TM (**Figure 1**): it consists of trabecular sheets that extend from the scleral spur to the lateral wall of the scleral groove.

    c. The juxtacanalicular TM (**Figure 1**): it forms the inner wall of the canal of Schlemm and the aqueous humor moves through and between the endothelial cells that line the inner wall of the canal of Schlemm. As we advance in these areas, the difficulty of the aqueous humor outflow increases, so it is believed that the juxtacanalicular TM is the main site of resistance to the outflow of the aqueous humor.

The TM is a pressure sensitive drainage site and acts as a one-way valve, regardless of the energy. Furthermore, its cells are phagocytic and can exhibit this function in the presence of inflammation and after laser trabeculoplasty [3].

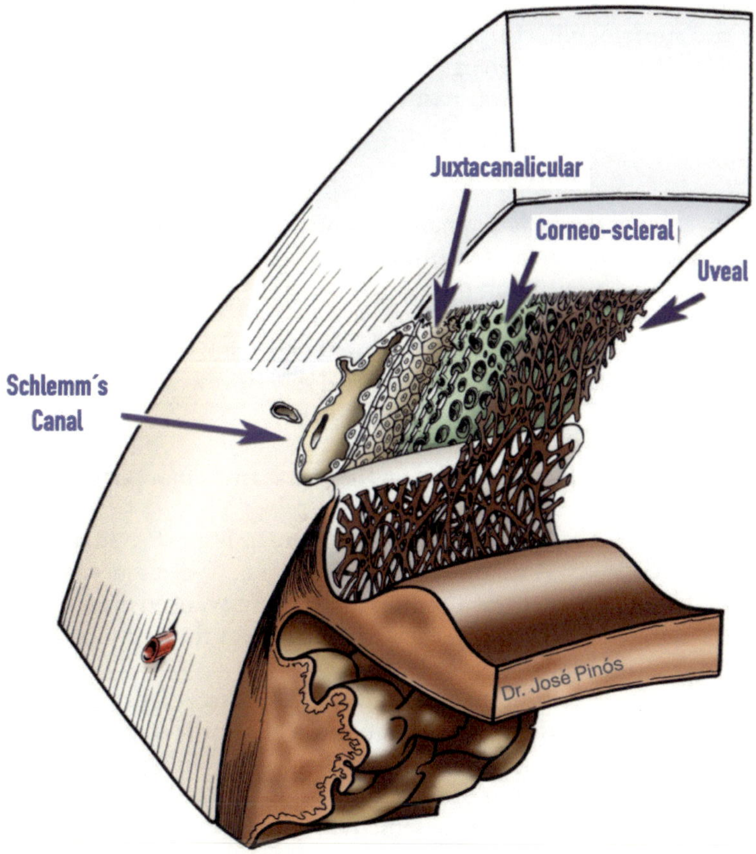

Figure 1.
Trabecular meshwork (uveal, corneo-scleral and juxtacanalicular); Schlemm's canal.

We should not understand this system as a succession of static networks. We should understand it as a tissue embedded in an extracellular matrix in which there is a continuous intra and extracellular filtration towards the Schlemm's canal (SC), in which there is a progressive deterioration in the case of eyes with glaucoma. Thus, in eyes with glaucoma, there are some alterations that will produce rigidity of this tissue difficulting the drainage of the aqueous humor.

2. The SC (**Figure 1**) is a single canal that surrounds the anterior chamber 360° and has a diameter of 200–300 μm [3]. SC is lined with an endothelial layer that rests on a discontinuous basement membrane [3]. It is not a homogeneous or rigid conduit. Microscopically it is a complex structure, as it is crossed by tubules and has partitions and duplications and has some structures such as cylindrical anchoring structures that communicate the trabecular face with the mouth of the collecting tubules that perform a valve-like function [3]. The outer wall of the Schlemm's canal is made up of single-layered cells of endothelium without pores [3]. With OCT we can also appreciate how the canal and the trabecular meshwork modifies with changes in IOP [4].

3. Finally we have the complex formed by the collectors, venous plexuses and the aqueous veins [3]. It is a complex system of vessels with abundant arteriovenous anastomoses, in which the transmission of the heartbeat is essential, and whose function is to carry the aqueous humor from SC to the systemic

circulation (it connects SC with the episcleral veins, that drain into the anterior and superior ciliary ophthalmic veins, which drain into the cavernous sinus) [3]. The organization of the collectors is not homogeneous, since they are mainly found in the lower nasal area.

In summary:

- The trabecular pathway is a dynamic tissue that has a pumping system towards the systemic circulation and is influenced by IOP changes (especially blinking, ocular pulse, eye movements).

- In glaucoma there are some ultrastructural alterations that will produce a loss of elasticity of the trabecular pathway and therefore a decrease in aqueous humor filtration.

- These changes are more important in the juxtacanalicular portion of the TM.

- It is logical that the trabecular pathway is more or less affected depending on the type of glaucoma. A mild, incipient glaucoma, with a few years of evolution, will have less structural alterations than an advanced glaucoma, with more years of evolution and that requires 2–3 drugs for its control.

- In the same way, the different anatomical alterations will produce a greater or lesser alteration of the TM. For example, a glaucoma that does not present any alteration in gonioscopy is different than a pseudoexfoliative glaucoma, in which the pigment enters in the TM and the rest of the angular structures, or a pigment dispersion glaucoma, in which the pigment permeates very intensively the entire TM.

3. Types of migs techniques in the trabecular pathway

All the surgical routes of the trabecular route seek the same aim (to facilitate the exit of aqueous humor from the anterior chamber to the systemic circulation) but they achieve it in different ways.

a. Some techniques perform microperforations, either with an implant (iStent) or with a laser (ELT).

b. Others perform a rupture of the internal wall of the shlemm canal and the trabecular meshwork (trabectome, Kahook, OMNI).

c. Others perform a viscodilation of the SC, leading to the distension of the Schlemm canal, of the trabecular meshwork and of the collecting canals (ABiC, OMNI).

We can also differentiate the surgeries based on the area that they treat:

a. Some provide a punctual treatment (iStent).

b. Others treat a sector, normally 90° (ELT, trabectome, Kahook).

c. Others treat the entire circumference (360°) of the SC (OMNI, ABiC, GATT).

Some of these techniques are detailed below.

3.1 iStent

3.1.1 Definition

It is an ab-interno MIGS technique in which two implants are applied in a specific way on the TM [5]. IStent is the smallest device ever implanted in humans [5]. It is a titanium implant surrounded by a layer of heparin, which allows better passage of the aqueous humor through the lumen of the iStent [5]. It has a long portion that enters the Schlemm's canal and a short portion that crosses the TM and connects with the anterior chamber [5]. The distal portion is beveled and tapered to facilitate penetration through the TM tissue and on the external surface it has three ridges that prevent its expulsion once inserted [5]. The Glaukos® GTS-400 trabecular implant has an applicator and a button to release the device and comes preloaded with two iStent, allowing the implantation of both iStent with a single applicator [5].

3.1.2 Indications and contraindications

This implant is ideal for surgery combined with phacoemulsification, since the angle is easier to visualize in pseudophakic eyes [5]. Thus, IStent is indicated in combined use with cataract surgery for reduction of IOP in adult patients with mild–moderate open angle glaucoma (OAG) under treatment with topical hypotensive drugs and cataract in surgical stage [5].

It is contraindicated in patients with both primary and secondary angle closure glaucoma, including neovascular glaucoma, as well as in patients with retrobulbar tumors, thyroid orbitopathy, Sturge–Weber Syndrome or any other situation that may cause elevated episcleral venous pressure [5].

A gonioscopy should be performed prior to surgery to exclude peripheral anterior synechiae, rubeosis or any other abnormality of the chamber angle that may hinder a correct visualization of the angle that could produce a possible incorrect placement of the iStent [5].

3.1.3 Surgical technique

For a safe surgery, it is essential to obtain a good visualization of the chamber angle by turning the patient's head 45° towards the opposite side of the operated eye and tilting the head of the surgical microscope 30° [5]. Intracamerular acetylcholine injection is first performed to constrict the pupil and the anterior chamber (AC) is filled with cohesive viscoelastic [5]. The main incision made for phacoemulsification is used to introduce the implant through the AC into the TM, while viewing the angle with gonioscopy and, once the insertion site is located, the tip of the implant (bevelled) is inserted into the TM, at an angle of about 15°, which facilitates penetration into the tissue, with the iStent tip pointing towards the patient's feet [4]. When it is verified that the TM covers the entire implant, it is released with the button of the applicator [5]. A small backflow of blood from the SC is frequent and reflects the proper position of the iStent [5]. Finally, the applicator is removed, the viscoelastic is washed and the corneal incision is sealed by hydrating the stroma [4]. In **Figure 2(A)** we can see two iStent correctly implanted in the TM.

3.1.4 Security

Trabecular stent implantation is a safe procedure with limited complications and no severe adverse events [5]. The most common of complications is implant obstruction and malposition [5]. The appearance of minimal hyphema during surgery is a sign of correct implant placement [5].

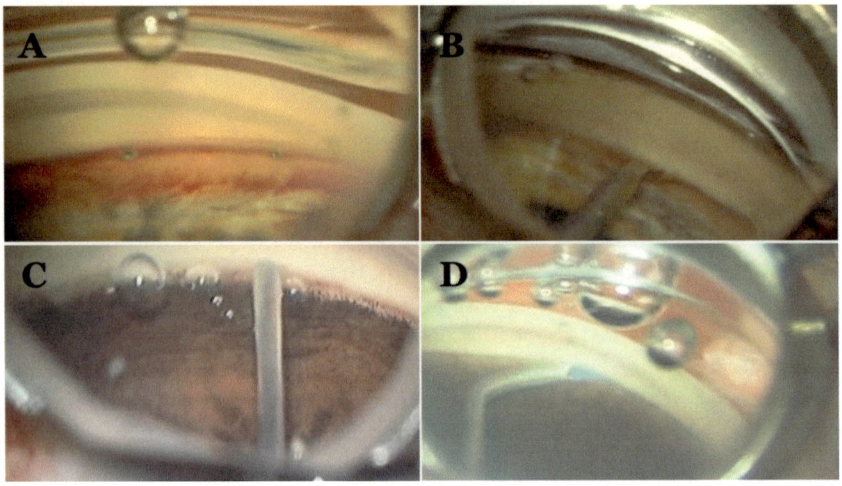

Figure 2.
Surgical procedures. (A) Two iStent correctly implanted in the TM. (B) Kahook mades a cut along the TM in a clockwise direction, followed by another cut in an anti-clockwise direction. (C) During the application of the laser in ELT, the whitening of the TM and the appearance of one or more bubbles are observed. (D) OMNI introduces the blue microcatheter in the SC, first for 180º of the SC and then the process is repeated for the second 180º.

3.2 ELT

3.2.1 Definition

ELT is an ab-interno MIGS technique in which microperforations or trabeculostomies are performed in the TM in order to facilitate the drainage of aqueous humor towards the SC using excimer laser impacts in a sectorial way (90°) of the TM [5]. Excimer laser photocoagulation allows the ablation of the juxtacanalicular wall of the TM and the internal wall of the Schlemm canal (avoiding injury to the external wall of the Schlemm canal containing fibroblasts, whose preservation is important for the drainage of the aqueous humor) with local and adjacent temperature control avoiding thermal damage to surrounding tissues [5].

3.2.2 Indications and contraindications

The effectiveness of ELT is greater when performed in combination with cataract surgery [6]. Therefore, it is indicated alone or in combination with cataract surgery in most patients with OAG with hypotensive treatment and cataract in surgical stage to reduce IOP and medication [5].

It is not indicated in glaucomas with increased episcleral venous pressure or in those requiring very low target IOPs below episcleral venous pressure [5].

3.2.3 Surgical technique

The AC is filled with viscoelastic using the corneal incision made for cataract surgery and the probe is positioned in contact with the TM, which can be visualized by gonioscopy (**Figure 2(C)**) or by endoscopy, depending on the generation of the laser used [5]. Between 8 and 10 laser microperforations are made per 90° sector of the TM [5]. The parameters used by the laser are: 200 μm spot, 1.2 mJ pulse energy, 80 ns duration [5]. During the application of the laser, the whitening of the TM and the appearance of one or more bubbles are observed.

(**Figure 2(C)**), sometimes associated with a slight reflux of blood that confirms the opening of the SC [5]. Finally, the probe is removed, the viscoelastic is washed, and the corneal incision is sealed by hydrating the stroma [5].

3.2.4 Security

This is a simple technique with a low incidence of complications. The main complications include hemorrhage in the immediate postoperative period and the fact that, due to the small size of the perforations, they are more easily obstructed than larger openings obtained with other procedures [5].

ELT can be performed on eyes that have previously undergone filtering surgery [5].

Its application in only 90° per session allows retreatment in the 3 remaining sectors in future interventions [5].

3.3 Kahook

3.3.1 Definition

It is a sectoral (90°) ab-interno MIGS technique in which the TM and the internal wall of the canal are bundled (similar to the procedure performed with the trabectome) with a device that is inserted into the TM and consists of a ramp in the distal end that, as we advance in the cut, raises the TM tissue and directs it towards 2 blades at the ends of the ramp that allow the cutting and extraction of this tissue [5].

3.3.2 Indications and contraindications

Thanks to its approach, it can be easily combined with cataract surgery and the combination of both surgeries increases hypotensive efficacy [7, 8]. Therefore, it is indicated in different types of OAG (primary, secondary to pseudoexfoliation and pigment dispersion, corticosteroid and uveitic), with mild or moderate glaucoma damage in a stage prior to conventional surgery, combined with cataract surgery in patients with cataract in the surgical stage in whom a decrease in IOP and/or a reduction in topical hypotensive medication is desired [5].

It should not be used in patients with advanced glaucoma or with a target IOP lower than episcleral venous pressure [5].

3.3.3 Surgical technique

The patient's head should be turned to the opposite side of the eye to be treated [5]. The corneal incision of cataract surgery is used to inject cohesive viscoelastic and introduce the kahook, which advances through the anterior chamber towards the nasal angle sector, which is visualized by gonioscopy [5]. The tip of the kahook is inserted through the TM into SC, and a cut is made along the TM in a clockwise direction, followed by another cut in an anti-clockwise direction, using the insertion site as a point of attachment reference (**Figure 2(B)**) [5]. The reflux of blood confirms the opening of the SC [5]. Finally, the device is removed, the viscoelastic is washed, and the corneal incision is sealed by hydrating the stroma [5].

3.3.4 Security

The complication rate is low and comparable to that of Trabectome™, highlighting the bleeding in the anterior chamber [9].

3.4 ABiC

3.4.1 Definition

Ab-interno canaloplasty (ABiC) is an ab-interno MIGS that viscodilate de TM, SC and the collerctor channels 360° inserting a microcatheter [10].

3.4.2 Indications and contraindications

ABiC is effective at reducing IOP and medication use in eyes with uncontrolled primary open-angle glaucoma (POAG) with or without cataract surgery [9]. It is useful in combination with cataract surgery as incisions resemble those of a typical cataract extraction and the IOP lowering effect of both procedures is enhanced [10]. Moreover, the addition of ABiC to phacoemulsification could be considered astigmatically neutral [10].

As in the resto of MIGS, the epiescleral venous-resistant floor limits the IOP-lowering effect, so ABiC seems to be indicated such as a minimal invasive technique that does not affect future conjunctival bleb surgeries in patients with or without cataracts and POAG that need a modest IOP-lowering effect in order to reduce IOP or medication [10].

3.4.3 Surgical technique

After cataract surgery, the side port corneal incision is used in order to introduce viscoelastic and the microcatheter towards the nasal angle [10]. A side port incision for the iTrack™ microcatheter is created approximately 90° away from de nasal drainage angle, wich is inserted into the AC with te catheter tip guided towards the nasal angle [10]. A 25 G needle or a Cystotome® is used to perform a micro-goniotomy in the nasal TM under visualization using a gonioprism [9]. The microcatheter is held by a micro-surgical forceps and the SC is intubated inserting the catheter through the goniotomy until complete the circumferential intubation of SC 360° [10]. After that, the catheter is slowly withdrawn while infusing viscoelastic every clock hour [9]. Finally, the catether is removed, the viscoelastic is washed, and the corneal incision is sealed by hydrating the stroma [10].

3.4.4 Security

ABiC shows no serious adverse events and less complications compared to more invasive conventional techniques; adverse events are limited to intraoperative bleeding at the goniotomy site and postoperative microhyphema [10].

3.5 OMNI

3.5.1 Definition

OMNI™ Surgical System is an ab-interno MIGS that combines two functions into one device: microcatherization and vascodilation in up to 360° of the SC (open distal outflow pathway) and cutting of the TM (controlled and Customizable trabeculotomy that removes the resistance of the TM) using a single fully integrated handheld system [11]. The system has got a luer fitting that allows for efficient priming of the device with viscoelastic, a priming lock, a reservoir where microcatheter is retracted, the gears whose movilization with the finger facilitate microcatheter deployment and retraction, a cannula with a beleved tip that allows for precise acces to target tissues, viscoelastic fluid and a blue microcatheter.

3.5.2 Indications and contraindications

As other MIGS techniques, OMNI can be used isolated or easily in conjunction with cataract surgery, in mild or moderated POAG that do not require a big IOP-lowering effect, with a minimal invasive approach and avoiding bleb complications and without conditioning future conjunctival bleb surgeries [11].

3.5.3 Surgical technique

The head of the patient and the microscope are tilted 30–40° and OMNI is introduced using the temporal clear corneal incision of the cataract surgery towards the nasal angle [11]. A small (<1 mm) goniotomy is created with the cannula tip in order to introduce the microcatheter for 180° of the SC under gonioscopic visualization (**Figure 2(D)**) [11]. Viscoelastic is delivered for viscodilation while microcatheter is retracted [11]. Microcatheter is again advanced and withdrawn with a 90° traction causing the unroof the SC (trabeculotomy) [11]. The process is repeated for the second 180° [10]. This technique allows varying the intensity of the treatment: for example, we can perform a 360° viscodylation and a 180° trabeculotomy.

3.5.4 Security

Adverse events are generally mild, nonseriuous and transient and include anterior chamber inflammation, posterior capsular opaciticity, IOP > 10 mmHg above baseline more than 30 days postoperatively, cystoid macular edema, corneal edema and hyphema [11].

4. Scientific evidence

Some techniques perform a more aggressive treatment than others. It is logical to think that the less aggressive techniques will be used in eyes with glaucoma where the involvement of the TM is smaller, and that, on the contrary, the more aggressive techniques, such as the trabeculotomy with viscodilatation, will be used in cases where the involvement of the TM is much more intense.

If we review the literature in order to compare the different surgical techniques [12–21], we see that, except in some surgical techniques, in the most of the techniques, most of the studies present biases: they are not randomized, they are not prospective, they are simple series, they do not have washout, they use personal criteria, they do not record complications ... therefore, we can affirm that the scientific evidence for MIGS surgery in comparison with other techniques is very limited, although it has been demonstrated a decrease in IOP, a decrease in the number of drugs and a decrease in complications.

If we focus on surgical success, understanding it such as a IOP reduction greater than 20%, most techniques reach a rate success of 60–80% (**Table 1**). Evidence A and B can only be found with the iStent, the Hydrus and the trabectome, while in OMNI and Kahook the grade of recommendation is C (**Table 1**).

If we focus on the IOP that these surgical techniques achieve, we see that in the most of the cases the IOP reached is between 15 and 17 mmHg (**Table 2**), a limitation that is given by the episcleral venous pressure.

iStent + cataract iStent + cataract	66% (12 M) 45% (24 M)	
iStent inject + cataract iStent inject	76% (12 M) 88% (12 M)	A
Hydrus + cataract Hydrus + cataract	88% (12 M) 80% (24 M)	A-B
Trabectome Trabectome + cataract	61% (12 M) 85% (24 M)	B
ABiC ABiC + cataract	82% (12 M) 88% (12 M)	C
Trab 360 OMNI OMNI + cataract	87% (12 M) 68% (12 M) 87% (12 M)	C
Kahook + cataract Kahook + cataract	57% (12 M) 69% (35 M)	C
ELT ELT + cataract	52% (24 M) 91% (12 M)	C
JM Navarro. MIGS trabeculares. Evidencia científica. SEO 2019.		

Table 1.
Surgical success achieved with different MIGS techniques.

Trabectome	16 mmHg	
Kahook	15 mmHg	16 mmHg
iStent Inject	17 mmHg	
Hydrus	17 mmHg	
ABiC	15 mmHg	
OMNI	16 mmHg	
ELT	16 mmHg	
JM Navarro. MIGS trabeculares. Evidencia científica. SEO 2019.		

Table 2.
IOP achieved with different MIGS techniques.

5. Conclusion

Taking all together, we can conclude with the following question: what can we expect from trabecular MIGS?

- MIGS are surgeries with a short learning technique, little aggressive and with a fast execution.
- They have few and little severe complications.
- They do not influence the possibility of performing surgeries with conjunctival bleb in the future if required.
- If we focus on the results, we will have a decrease greater than 20% in almost two thirds of surgeries, with a decrease of one or two drugs.

- However, the target pressure they achieve is approximately 16 mmHg. This means that they can be useful in eyes with mild or moderate glaucoma that do not require a big IOP decrease, but that in eyes with advanced glaucoma, where we look forward an IOP below 15 mmHg, trabecular MIGS techniques are not the most appropriate.

Author details

Marina Aguilar González*, Jorge Vila Arteaga and Jose Marí Cotino
Hospital Universitario y Politécnico la Fe, Calle Fernando Abril Martorell, 106, 16026, Valencia, Spain

*Address all correspondence to: aguilarmarina.oft@gmail.com

References

[1] Poley BJ, Lindstrom RL, Samuelson TW, Schulze R Jr. Intraocular pressure reduction after phacoemulsification with intraocular lens implantation in glaucomatous and nonglaucomatous eyes: evaluation of a causal relationship between the natural lens and open-angle glaucoma. Journal of Cataract and Refractive Surgery. 2009;**35**:1946-1955

[2] Mansberger SL. A need for glaucoma surgery (with o without cataract). American Academy Ophthalmology: The case for cataract surgery alone. Subespeciality day Glaucoma; 2012

[3] Christopher A Girkin MD, Chair AMB, MD JGC, MBBS PD, Giaconi JAA, MD FAM, et al. Section 10: Glaucoma. In: American Academy of Ophthalmology (AAO). 2018

[4] Gillmann K, Bravetti GE, Mermoud A, Mansouri K. A Prospective Analysis of iStent Inject Microstent Positioning: Schlemm Canal Dilatation and Intraocular Pressure Correlations. Journal of Glaucoma. 2019 Jul;**28**(7):613-621

[5] Cosme Lvin Dapena, Pablo Alcocer Yuste. Cirugía microincisional del glaucoma. N°1 edición. Sociedad Española de Oftalomología (SEO). 2016.

[6] Francis BA, Singh K, Lin SC, Hodapp E, Jampel HD, Samples JR, et al. Novel glaucoma procedures: a report by the American Academy of Ophthalmology. Ophthalmology. 2011;**118**(7):1466-1480

[7] Francis BA. Trabectome combined with phacoemulsification versus phacoemulsification alone: a prospective, nonrandomized, controlled trial. Clinical & Surgical Ophthalmology. 2010;**28**:10

[8] Francis BA, Winarko S. Combined Trabectome and cataract surgery versus combined trabeculectomy and cataract surgery in open-angle glaucoma. Clinical & Surgical Ophthalmology. 2011;**29**:2/3

[9] Nakasato H, Uemoto R, Isozaki M, Meguro A, Kawagoe T, Mizuki N. Trabeculotomy ab interno with internal limiting membrane forceps for open-angle glaucoma. Graefe's Archive for Clinical and Experimental Ophthalmology. 2014;**252**(6):977-982

[10] Gallardo MJ, Supnet RA, Ahmed IIK. Viscodilation of Schlemm's canal for the reduction of IOP via an ab-interno approach. Clinical Ophthalmology. 2018;**23**(12):2149-2155

[11] Vold SD, Williamson BK, Hirsch L, Aminlari AE, Cho AS, Nelson C, Dickerson JE Jr. Canaloplasty and Trabeculotomy with the OMNI System in Pseudophakic Patients with Open-Angle Glaucoma: The ROMEO Study. Ophthalmol Glaucoma. 2020:S2589-4196(20)30264-7.

[12] Samuelson TW, Sarkisian SR Jr, Lubeck DM, Stiles MC, Duh YJ, Romo EA, Giamporcaro JE, Hornbeak DM, Katz LJ; iStent inject Study Group. Prospective, Randomized, Controlled Pivotal Trial of an Ab Interno Implanted Trabecular Micro-Bypass in Primary Open-Angle Glaucoma and Cataract. Two-Year Results. Ophthalmology. 2019;**126**(6):811-821

[13] Craven ER, Katz LJ, Wells JM, Giamporcaro JE, iStent Study Group. Cataract surgery with trabecular micro-bypass stent implantation in patients with mild-to-moderate open-angle glaucoma and cataract: two-year follow-up. Journal of Cataract and Refractive Surgery. 2012;**38**(8):1339-1345

[14] Samuelson TW, Sarkisian SR Jr, Lubeck DM, Stiles MC, Duh YJ, Romo EA, Giamporcaro JE, Hornbeak DM, Katz LJ; iStent inject Study Group. Prospective, Randomized, Controlled Pivotal Trial of an Ab Interno Implanted Trabecular Micro-Bypass in Primary Open-Angle Glaucoma and Cataract. Two-Year Results. Ophthalmology. 2019;**126**(6):811-821

[15] Fea AM, Belda JI, Rękas M, Jünemann A, Chang L, Pablo L, et al. Prospective unmasked randomized evaluation of the iStent inject (®) versus two ocular hypotensive agents in patients with primary open-angle glaucoma. Clinical Ophthalmology. 2014;**8**:875-882

[16] Pfeiffer N, Garcia-Feijoo J, Martinez-de-la-Casa JM, Larrosa JM, Fea A, Lemij H, et al. Randomized Trial of a Schlemm's Canal Microstent with Phacoemulsification for Reducing Intraocular Pressure in Open-Angle Glaucoma. Ophthalmology. 2015;**122**(7):1283-1293

[17] Gallardo MJ, Supnet RA, Ahmed IIK. Viscodilation of Schlemm's canal for the reduction of IOP via an ab-interno approach. Clinical Ophthalmology. 2018;**23**(12):2149-2155

[18] Dorairaj SK, Seibold LK, Radcliffe NM, Aref AA, Jimenez-Román J, Lazcano-Gomez GS, et al. 12-Month Outcomes of Goniotomy Performed Using the Kahook Dual Blade Combined with Cataract Surgery in Eyes with Medically Treated Glaucoma. Advances in Therapy. 2018;**35**(9):1460-1469

[19] Pache M, Wilmsmeyer S, Funk J. Laserchirurgie und Glaukom: Excimer-Laser-Trabekulotomie [Laser surgery for glaucoma: excimer-laser trabeculotomy]. Klinische Monatsblätter für Augenheilkunde. 2006;**223**(4):303-307

[20] Pache M, Wilmsmeyer S, Funk J. Laserchirurgie und Glaukom: Excimer-Laser-Trabekulotomie [Laser surgery for glaucoma: excimer-laser trabeculotomy]. Klinische Monatsblätter für Augenheilkunde. 2006;**223**(4):303-307

[21] Babighian S, Caretti L, Tavolato M, Cian R, Galan A. Excimer laser trabeculotomy vs 180 degrees selective laser trabeculoplasty in primary open-angle glaucoma. A 2-year randomized, controlled trial. Eye (London, England). 2010;**24**(4):632-638

Chapter 3

Cataract Surgery in Post-Vitrectomized Eyes

Olivia Esteban, Javier Mateo, Paula Casas, Javier Lara and Javier Ascaso

Abstract

Because of the application of vitreoretinal surgical techniques to a broader range of posterior segment diseases and because cataract develops frequently in postvitrectomy eyes, cataract surgeons should be familiar with the challenges of cataract extraction in vitrectomized eyes. Cataract surgery after pars plana vitrectomy significantly improves visual acuity in 85% of cases, limited by retinal comorbidity and surgical complications. However, despite recent advances, this surgery remains a special challenge. The cataract surgeon can prepare for these challenges with awareness of such potential factors as an excessively mobile posterior capsule, silicon oil removal and special considerations concerning intraocular lens selection and power calculation. And consider the postoperative complications as posterior capsule opacification or refractive errors.

Keywords: cataract, intraocular lens, vitrectomy

1. Introduction

Pars plana vitrectomy is a surgical technique that allows a successful treatment of many diseases of the posterior segment of the eye, such as retinal detachment, proliferative diabetic retinopathy, vitreous hemorrhage, epiretinal membrane, or macular hole, among others. The increase in vitreoretinal surgery procedures has led to a predictable and consequent increase in cataract surgery in these eyes. Therefore, the ophthalmologist must be aware of the special characteristics of this type of patient and the impact of a vitrectomized eye on cataract surgery.

2. Development of cataract

Cataract formation or progression is one of the most frequent complications we can find after vitreoretinal surgery. According to several studies, up to 65–80% of the eyes develop a cataract in the 24 months following vitrectomy. [1–6]

Although posterior subcapsular and cortical cataracts can be formed after surgery especially in young patients, nuclear cataracts are much more frequent. Transient subcapsular opacification in the early postoperative period is not unusual. The time interval between vitrectomy and phacoemulsification can vary between 9 and 29 months. [1–3, 7–12]

Even though the exact etiology of cataracts formed after vitrectomy is not known, there are several elements that seem to have a role in it as predisposing or precipitating factors:

- Age: patients over 50 years of age show a significant increase in cataract incidence after retinal surgery when compared to younger ones. They usually develop a nuclear sclerosis, whereas posterior subcapsular opacification is more usual at earlier ages. Whenever there is a previous cataract, vitrectomy favors its progression. [1, 2, 8, 13–15]

- Composition of fluid infusion into the vitreous cavity: the high concentration of 150 mmHg of oxygen in the irrigating solutions used during vitrectomy, much higher than the 17 mmHg of the anterior vitreous or the 30 mmHg of the aqueous, may contribute to the oxidation of the proteins of the lens, thus accelerating the formation of cataracts. However, it remains to be demonstrated that this exposure to high levels of oxygen is maintained in the postoperative period. [2, 15–17]

- Diabetes: there seems to be a lower rate of cataract progression in vitrectomized diabetics (especially in cases of ischemic retinopathy) compared to patients without diabetes, given that the oxygen level in their vitreous is lower (**Figure 1**). [18, 19]

- Direct surgical damage: iatrogenic cataracts can be generated by direct trauma to the posterior lens capsule from the instruments used during pars plana vitrectomy, causing its rupture and producing a very rapid lens opacification. Trauma is more likely to be suffered in long difficult surgeries, such as retinal detachment with vitreoretinal proliferation. If a cataract is formed in the four months following retinal surgery, traumatic etiology should be suspected. [1, 20]

- Light toxicity: intense exposure to surgical microscope light or the fiber optic probe can be a factor that facilitates the oxidative damage of lens proteins. However, light sources currently incorporate Xenon light filter systems that eliminate the phototoxic fraction of the blue-ultraviolet wavelength, reducing the phototoxicity caused in the lens or in the retina. [2]

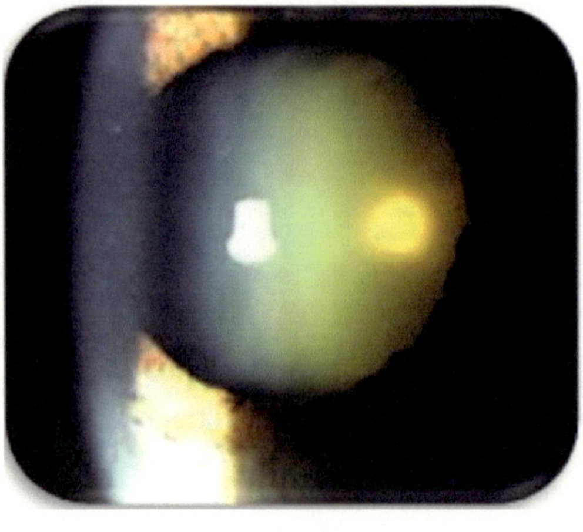

Figure 1.
Development of a nuclear cataract in a diabetic patient after six months of vitrectomy.

- Vitreous gel removal: the elimination of the vitreous seems to increase the level of retrolental oxygen, generating oxidation of the lens proteins. The incidence of cataracts is much higher after an extensive removal of the vitreous gel and it drops significantly when a limited vitrectomy or a nonvitrectomizing technique is performed. In other surgical procedures that do not include vitrectomy, such a scleral buckling or pneumatic retinopexy, the risk of inducing cataracts is also lower. [1, 2, 6, 17, 21, 22]

- Vitreous substitutes: the presence of gas bubble (SF6 or C3F8) or silicone oil in the vitreous chamber raise the incidence of lens opacification when compared with eyes without any tamponade after surgery. Long lasting substances increase even more the cataract progression. Lens opacity in patients with silicone oil is associated with epithelial cell metaplasia due to inhibition of lens metabolism (anaerobic glycolysis). Secondary gas-related lens opacities can appear as posterior subcapsular vacuoles, which sometimes can be transient and disappear if a layer of liquid is maintained between the gas bubble and the posterior surface of the lens. It is important for the patient to keep the head in a prone position, to prevent the meniscus of the gas bubble from contacting the posterior surface of the lens, and to avoid metabolic disruption of the lens cells. [1, 2, 8]

- Small gauge vitrectomy: although theoretically one of the advantages of the minimally invasive vitreo retinal surgery (23, 25 or 27 gauge) was the lower incidence of cataracts following the operation, there are no studies that demonstrate this relationship. No significant differences have been found between the different systems in the rate of cataract development. It seems that the progression of the lens opacification depends more on the amount of vitreous gel removed rather than the size of the instruments that are used. [1, 23–25]

3. Considerations before cataract surgery

The surgical criteria should be early, avoiding advanced cataracts requiring higher ultrasound power or poor posterior pole exploration. The final visual acuity after retinal surgery and the underlying retinal pathology for which vitrectomy was required to predict the visual prognosis of the patient should be identified through the anamnesis: retinal detachment with or without macular involvement, proliferative diabetic retinopathy with or without macular edema, history of ocular trauma or high myopia, among others. At times, it is difficult to determine whether the degree of visual impairment in the patient is due to underlying retinal pathology or to cataract progression. In patients operated on for macular disease who present metamorphopsia or central scotoma, these symptoms will persist after cataract surgery. Likewise, it is important to identify the time interval between vitrectomy and cataract, since when opacity occurs at intervals of less than 4 months, iatrogenic lens touch in the posterior capsule must be ruled out. [20]

In the ophthalmological examination, pupillary dilation should be evaluated, as in uveitic or diabetic eyes, and the state of the zonular fibers, since there may be phacoiridodonesis due to alteration of the zonule in vitrectomized eyes. It is important to perform a fundus examination to rule out retinal pathology and, occasionally, to perform an optical coherence tomography (OCT) to assess the status of the macula. In patients with macular edema, the need to treat it with an intravitreal injection before surgery or during the procedure itself will be assessed. In the case of not being able to visualize the fundus, an ocular ultrasound should be performed to assess the state of the retina and be able to rule out complications such as vitreous hemorrhage or retinal detachment that require combined surgery.

4. Intraocular lens calculation

Intraocular lens power calculation is based on the measurement of anatomical eye parameters. Regardless of the formula we apply, to calculate the intraocular lens (IOL) in our patients we must know precisely the axial length (AL), keratometry and anterior chamber depth (ACD). Prediction of IOL power in eyes undergoing retinal surgery can sometimes be challenging and certain considerations should be taken into account.

4.1 Axial length measurement

AL in our patients can be quantified using optical or ultrasonic methods. Optical methods are more comfortable because they do not require contact with the patient and are more examiner-independent. However, there are cases where we will turn to ultrasonic methods, especially because of media opacity.

Measuring AL requires proper foveal fixation, this could be an important source and error in patients with retinal pathologies. [26, 27] Newly developed equipment such as the IOL master 700, incorporates an OCT system to ensure a correct measurement aligned with the patient's fovea [27] this is especially important in cases of macular pathology and staphyloma. [28]

4.2 Axial length in vitrectomized eyes

In vitrectomized patients with no fluid exchange the vitreous is replaced by aqueous humor. This is not a problem with ultrasonic biometry because of the transmission rate of aqueous and vitreous humors are practically the same (1532 m/sec ultrasound velocity). In the same way, the vitreous has an optical refractive index of 1.3346 and the aqueous of 1.3336. This small difference generates a myopic shift of −0.13 diopters (D) in vitrectomized eyes that has little clinical relevance. [29, 30]

Ultrasound biometry measures AL from corneal vortex to internal limiting membrane along the optical axis. Optical systems quantify AL from corneal vortex to retinal pigment epithelium along visual axis. [31] So, macular status as macular edema or submacular fluid can affect the measurement of axial length in ultrasonic biometry. The difference in measurement with respect to the axis confers superiority to the optical biometer, which achieves more accurate measurements as long as the visual fixation of the patient is preserved to look at the laser target. [32]

Elevated myopia or staphyloma are more common in vitrectomized patients. [33] These factors along with poor visual binding are frequent cause of erroneous AL measurements. It is likely that one of the most complex situations to determine AL is the case of high retinal detachment with macula-off, where the patient cannot fix and foveal detachment generates an underestimation of AL. [34]

4.3 Axial length in oil-filled eyes

Phacoemulsification and silicone oil (SO) removal in a single act could avoid surgical risks and is optimal for patients with cataract formation in a short time after vitrectomy with SO tamponade. Obtaining accurate AL measurements in silicone oil-filled eyes can be difficult.

Whenever possible, we should quantify the AL in oil-filled eyes with optical biometers (optical interferometry or reflectance) because of the optical laser is not appreciably affected by SO, by its molecular weight or by the interfaces that remain between aqueous humor and silicone in eyes with incomplete filling. [35, 36] In the main menu of our optical biometer we will select the option "vitreous cavity filled with oil" and the refractive index of light will change from 1.33 in vitreous to 1.4 in silicone oil (**Figure 2**). [37]

However, cataracts generated by silicone oil are often dense and do not allow optical biometrics to be performed. It is estimated that in 4.7–17% of AL measurements, interferometry cannot be performed due to poor visual acuity, corneal opacity or dense cataract among others. [38, 39] Low coherence reflectometry and optical coherence tomography use longer wavelength than interferometry, so we can assume that the proportion of eyes measured with these techniques should be greater. [40] In cases where measurement with optical systems cannot be performed AL measurement becomes a biometric challenge.

The replacement of vitreous with silicone oil implies that the propagation of acoustic waves is modified. The speed of sound in a medium is inversely related to the refractive index of the medium. Because silicone has a higher rate than vitreous, it reduces the speed of sound a 36% approximately. The sound velocity declines from 1532 m/sec in the vitreous to 980 m/sec in 1000 centistokes molecular weight silicone oil. [41] This reduction in speed generates a higher axial length measurement. If we do not calibrate our ultrasonic biometer, we will generate a hypermetropic refractive defect.

If we use higher molecular weight silicone oil the speed variation would be different [42–45].

If our ultrasonic biometer does not have a speed adjustment for eyes with silicone oil, we can multiply a corrective factor of 0.64 to the vitreous cavity length obtained with a speed of 1532 m/sec. [46] To calculate the axial length we will have to add the rest of the structures (anterior chamber depth, lens thickness and retrosilicone space) to the value obtained from vitreous cavity with the corrective factor. [37]

Another source of error appears when the vitreous cavity is not completely filled with SO. An aqueous space is generated between the oil and the retina, the "retrosilicone space". It is maximum in supine position, decreases when the patient is erect and is minimized in the prone position. [47] And as we have seen before, it should

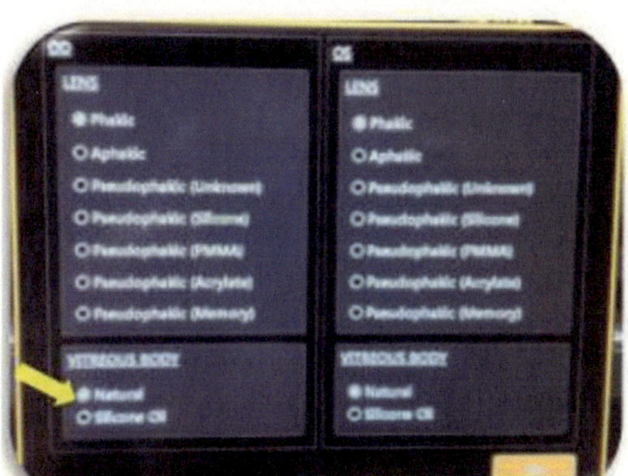

Figure 2.
Optical biometry and topography (Aladdin Topcon®). Select silicone oil in biometer before measuring AL.

be taken into account for IOL calculation. If we do not consider it, leads to a shorter and erroneous measurement of the AL in A-mode biometry.

Abu El Einen et al. [43] found better refractive results in oil-filled eyes explored by inmersion B-guided than in contact A-mode biometry. Although both are echographic techniques, immersion ultrasound prevents us from possible compression of the scanning probe on the cornea and mode B helps us to locate fovea, specially in patients with staphyloma or fluid interfaces. [48]

In addition to slower sound speed, SO absorbs sound, leading to poor penetration with low-quality echoes. [49] This significant sound attenuation generates poor identification of the retinal spike by contact A-mode biometry. [50] In these cases biometry may be unsatisfactory and other methods as we mention below have been proposed. Vitreoretinal surgeons should know that the appearance of cataract occurs after 3 months in 100% of the eyes with SO. [51, 52] Therefore, a useful strategy would be to perform a pre-vitrectomy biometry in all cases with macula on in which there is a possibility of fluid exchange by SO. [53] In these cases, we should take into account that the placement of a scleral buckle during surgery will also modify the axial length of the patient. [54, 55]

Another option is the two-step surgery with the removal of cataract and silicone oil in a first step and the placement of an implant in a second time if the retina remains stable. [56, 57]

El-Baha et al. perform more complex techniques with intraoperative biometry after remove SO with a sterilized ultrasonic biometer probe. [58] Elbendary et al. make an intraoperative calculation with a portable retinoscope. [59] These techniques consume more intraoperative time and require more specific devices that are not available in all centers, including a large stock of IOL powers.

4.4 Silicone oil refractive effect

In some patients, SO is not removed and is left inside the eye indefinitely. This is the case of eyes with recurrent bleeding or multiple retinal re-detachments among others. In this situation, if we want to extract the cataract we must take into account the refractive effect of SO when calculating IOL. SO acts as a negative lens because of its lower refractive index compared to vitreous. We must add +2 to +3 D to the calculated IOL to compensate for this effect, always in flat-convex lenses with the flat face toward the vitreous cavity. [60]

4.5 Changes in other eye parameters after vitrectomy

The anterior segment morphology has a crucial role for the refractive results after surgery. Moreover, calculation of effective lens position (ELP) in vitrectomized eyes is influenced by factors inherent to vitreous surgery.

The most uncertain factor in biometry after phaco-vitrectomy is postoperative ACD. Modification of ACD is controversial and there is no consensus on whether it increases or decreases. Mijnsbrugge et al. [61] reported a more posterior position of the IOL in the phacovitrectomy group compared to single phacoemulsification group, attributed to loss of vitreous support. Gülkilik, Neudorfer and Li [62–64] described no significant change in ACD postoperatively in phacovitrectomy group. And Hamoudi and Huang [65, 66] found an earlier position of IOL secondary to capsular fibrosis.

The influence of gas tamponade on refractive outcomes has also been studied, a myopic shift appears related to anterior lens displacement and shallower aqueous depth due to buoyancy and surface tension of the gas. [67] Even when the gas has already completely disappeared, it seems that the IOL could be fixed in a more anterior position. [67]

4.6 Lens calculation formulas in vitrectomized eyes

In recent years, the development of new biometric formulas to calculate the power of IOL to be implanted to our patients has allowed the minimization of post-surgical refractive surprises. New biometric calculation formulas use a variety of strategies, such as the inclusion of more predictive ELP values, the use of ray tracing, or artificial intelligence to achieve optimal post-surgical results.

There is currently no consensus on the most accurate method for biometric calculation in vitrectomized patients.

Lamson et al. [26] observed in a retrospective study that refractive outcomes using eight biometric formulas (Holladay 1, SRK/T, Barrett, Hill-radial basis function, Ladas and Holladay 2) were more variable and more hyperopic than in non-vitrectomized populations. The Holladay 2 formula obtained the highest percentages of postoperative refraction with predicted errors between ±0.50 D and ± 1 D. However, we should point out that the study was retrospective and analyzed a reduced sample of patients. In addition, there were important uncontrolled variables such as the implanted IOL model, which was not the same in all participants of the study. This hyperopic shift in vitrectomized eyes also was reported by Lee et al. [68]

Recently, another retrospective study published by Tan et al. [69] evaluated the refractive results obtained in cataract surgery in vitrectomized eyes by applying next-generation formulas (Barett Universal II, EVO, Kane, and Ladas super formula) against traditional formulas (Haigis, Hoffer Q, Holladay 1, and SRK/T) with Wang-Koch axial length adjustment if required. Before the lens constants were optimized, hyperopic outcomes were noted for all formulas, except for the Kane formula, which revealed no statistically significant bias. However, lens constant optimization enabled optimal and comparable results for all formulas.

As general recommendations to calculate IOL in vitrectomized eyes we suggest.

The optimization of the constant in clinical practice or, if not possible, choose a slightly myopic refractive target for the IOL to be implanted (−0.5 D).

Traditional formulas in miopic patients with axial length more than 26 mm should be used with Wang-Koch's correction.

The presence of silicone oil in the vitreous cavity does not change the choice of the biometric formula.

4.7 Considerations in combinated phaco-vitrectomy

Phaco-vitrectomy is mandatory in cases of retinal surgery with prior cataract. In addition, a large proportion of patients undergoing vitrectomy will develop cataract in the following years. Therefore, phaco-vitrectomy is a common procedure even without prior cataract as it saves costs and risks of a second intervention.

Unlike surgery in previously vitrectomized patients, where the tendency was to a hypocorrection after phacoemulsification (see "LENS CALCULATION FORMULAS IN VITRECTOMIZED EYES"). Phacoemulsification performed concurrently with vitrectomy seems to be associated with myopic shift in the refractive outcome [26, 34, 61, 70] Tranos et al. [70] found that postoperative refractive deviation greater than 0.5 D was associated with shallower ACD and increased macular thickness. Shiraki and Schweitzer [71, 72] related the myopic shift in combined phaco-vitrectomy with the gas tamponade commonly used in cases of retinal detachment. On the other hand, Vandergeest et al. [73] found no tendency toward a myopic shift and they got an elevated percentage of refractive accuracy in combined procedures.

Different from phacoemulsification in previously vitrectomized cases and faced with the variability of published results, our recommendation in cases of phaco-vitrectomy combined surgery would be to calculate the intraocular lens with a refractive target of zero.

5. Intraoperative complications

It has been reported that cataract extraction in eyes with previous vitrectomy is often more complicated because of various anatomic changes in the eye. In the vitrectomized eye, whose vitreous cavity was filled with air, gas or liquid solutions, the aqueous humor is the one that ends up occupying said space, so the lens does not have the counter pressure of the vitreous, which is a semi-solid and viscous substance, and during cataract surgery can occur significant variations in the depth of the anterior chamber that make the procedure difficult. Potential complications that may arise from this situation include bad pupil dilatation, zonule damage, posterior synechia, posterior capsule tears, increase mobility of complex lens-iris and altered intraocular fluid dynamics as a result of the absence of the anterior hyaloid face. Thus, cataract surgery (phacoemulsification) in vitrectomized eyes has been reported to be associated with an increased rate of complications. [74–77]

Cataract surgery in the vitrectomized eye can be performed under topical anesthesia, or in complex cases local anesthesia. When surgery was performed under topical anesthesia, the anterior chamber was irrigated with lidocaine 0.5% before it was filled with an ophthalmic viscosurgical device. There are ophthalmologists who prefer peri- or retrobulbar anesthesia, since when the anterior chamber is deepened, oscillations of the irido-crystalline diaphragm occur with variation in pupillary diameter that generates discomfort to the patient. If the surgery is performed using local anesthesia (retrobulbar), it is necessary to be cautious with the pressure exerted by the Honan balloon. Excessive pressure exerted by this balloon could damage or increase damage to a compromised zonule, increasing the risk of intraoperative drop of the nucleus into the vitreous cavity. For this reason, the use of topical anesthesia is preferable for cataract surgery in previously vitrectomized eyes. Finally, general anesthesia will be reserved for children, neurological and psychiatric patients and bad collaborators.

Biro et al. reported posterior capsule tears and dropped nucleus in 7,3% in 41 vitrectomized patiens. [78]

Nevertheless, others authors suggest that eyes with and without prior pars plana vitrectomy (PPV) have a similar likelihood of having intraoperative complications. These authors reported that recognize the differences in the physiologic state of the vitrectomized eye compared with that of non-vitrectomized eyes reduced the frequency of intraoperative complications. [79]

A clear corneal incision for performing the phacoemulsification was recommended, avoiding the conjuntival-scleral scarring from previous retinal surgery. [80]

No intraoperative wound-related problems have been described using this clear corneal approach, with a 3-step wound construction with a 50% vertical groove.

In patients with inadequate dilation of the pupil, the use of intracamerular phenylephrine or the insertion of iris retractors or pupillary elongation maneuvers will be evaluated, and if there are posterior synechiae, synechiolysis will be performed with the help of viscoelastics.

In the case of severe crystalline opacities that do not allow the visualization of the background orange reflex, the use of trypan blue in the staining of the anterior capsule, facilitating capsulorhexis, will be considered. In vitrectomized eyes, trypan blue must be introduced into the anterior chamber slowly to avoid its diffusion to the vitreous chamber through zonular dehiscences. If this happens, phacoemulsification can be very complicated by the loss of the foveal reflex, increasing the risk of rupture of the posterior capsule.

If possible, very small capsulorhexis should be avoided to avoid capsular phimosis that later hinders the evaluation of the retinal periphery. Both cohesive viscoelastics that have expansive property allowing the management of mydriasis, and dispersives that protect the corneal endothelium can be used.

Phacoemulsification with a constant pressure minimizes complications in the event of significant ocular collapse. [81]

Fluctuations in the anterior chamber, such as the antero and retropulsion phenomenon, can be minimized by keeping the infusion bottle low, although sometimes there are unavoidable intraoperative mioses that make surgery difficult.

Accurately sized wounds, including the clear corneal incision for the phaco tip and the side port for the nucleus manipulator, help to maintain a relatively sealed chamber during surgery and minimize fluctuation of the anterior chamber depth.

In the case of having a reverse pupillary blockage, produced when the iris contacts the anterior capsule, preventing the flow from reaching the posterior chamber, it can be solved either by lifting the iris with a second instrument from the paracentesis or using the phaco tip lifting the iris and put the foot pedal in the irrigation level before any phaco manipulation.

In a study of 75 vitrectomized eyes, this blockage was observed in 53.3% of the cases during cataract surgery, especially in younger patients, with greater axial length and greater anterior chamber depth. [82]

Infusion deviation syndrome occurs when fluid migrates backward through the zonule and it increases the volume of the vitreous and causes flattening of the anterior chamber. Titiyal et al. [83] presented this complication in 12.3% of the 89 vitrectomized eyes during cataract surgery. To prevent this, it is recommended to carry out the hydration maneuvers carefully, reduce the flow of fluid within the anterior chamber (lowering the height of the bottles if possible or reducing the flow/aspiration rate). Once this complication appears, it is very useful to place in the pars plana a vitrectomy trocar without a valve to allow the pressure to escape from the posterior chamber and to be able to continue performing phacoemulsification.

Maneuvers that push the lens during phacoemulsification and cause zonular tension should be avoided. Thorough careful hydrodissection, confirmation of adequate lens rotation before phacoemulsification and gentle nucleus manipulation help to avoid unnecessary zonular damage and posterior capsule tears. If there is a fall of the nucleus or fragments to the vitreous cavity after the rupture of the posterior capsule, aggressive maneuvers should not be carried out when trying to recover them since they can generate ruptures in the retina and subsequent retinal detachment. The appropriate management in these cases is to perform a posterior approach to the complication through pars plana vitrectomy. In general, it is recommended to complete the vitrectomy if necessary, ensure by direct visualization that retinal tears have not been generated, removal of all fragments (either using the vitreotome or using the posterior chamber phacoemulsifier). In these cases, exploration of the peripheral retina to detect tears by indentation is highly recommended (**Figures 3** and **4**).

If there is good capsular support, a lens can be placed in the capsular bag remnants or in the sulcus if the anterior capsule remains intact. In the latter case, it is highly recommended to perform the Gimbel maneuver, which consists of dislocating the optic of the intraocular lens through the opening of the anterior capsule, keeping the haptics of the lens in sulcus. With this maneuver great stability in the implanted intraocular lens is obtained. The technique provides stability and

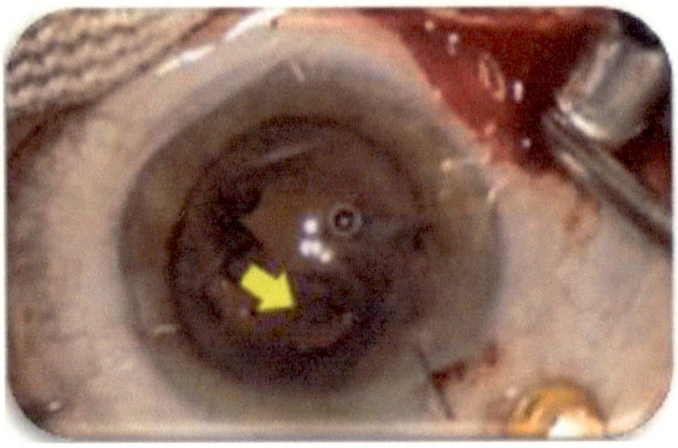

Figure 3.
Posterior capsule tear (yellow arrow) in a post-vitrectomized cataract surgery.

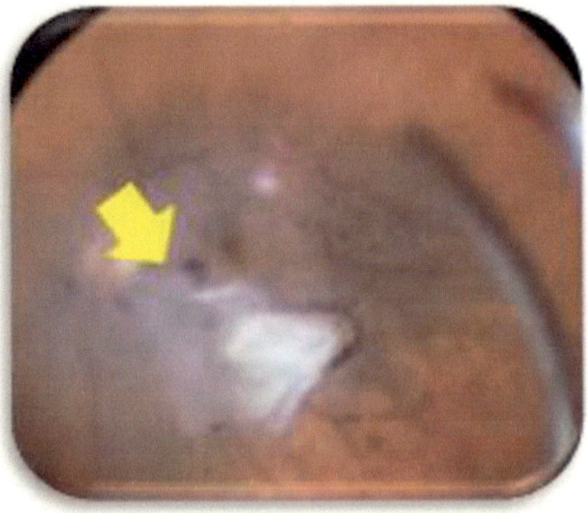

Figure 4.
Subluxated fragments of the lens (yellow arrow) to the retina in a complicated post-vitrectomized cataract surgery.

long-term centration of the IOL and prevents vitreous from extending anterior to the IOL. [84]

If there is no capsular support, other alternatives must be chosen to place the intraocular lens, such as the sulcus-sutured lens or the iris fixation lenses.

The use of multifocal lenses in eyes with retinal pathology remains controversial, so it is generally preferred to implant single vision lenses.

6. Postoperative complications

Vitrectomized patients after cataract surgery have a higher risk of postoperative complications. In patients with previous macular surgery and diabetic eyes, a higher incidence of cystic macular edema has been observed. It was reported after a mean time of 42 days after cataract surgery. [85] Nevertheles, there are other studies which have not found CME however, OCT was not routinely used. Therefore, it is important to monitor these patients with fundus and OCT postoperatively since some are refractory cases and require subtenon or intravitreal treatment (**Figure 5**). [86, 87]

Patients with a history of retinal detachment or high myopia surgery may have a higher incidence of retinal detachment, so the peripheral retina should be evaluated throughout the postoperative period. The incidence of RD has been reported between 2% and 8% in different studies [88–90]. Cataract surgery in these patients

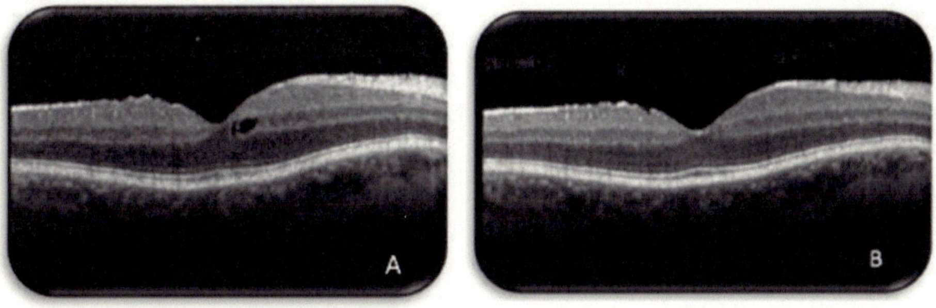

Figure 5.
Asymptomatic cystic macular edema four weeks after cataract surgery in a vitrecomized patient (A). Resolution of macular cystics after topical non-steroidal anti-inflammatory treatment (B).

can no have intra-operative complication which may predispose to RD. Therefore, this complication was a consequence of the previous posterior segment pathology in these eyes.

The incidence of posterior capsular opacification (PCO) was higher in vitrectomized eyes compared with nonvitrectomized eyes. [91, 92] It is ranging between 2.2% and 19.9% [15–17] within the first year after surgery. [88–90].

Finally, another complication in vitrectomized patients undergoing cataract surgery may be long-term subluxations or dislocations of the lens to the vitreous cavity. High myopia was the most frequent predisposing factor in 18.1% of the 83 eyes with this complication. [93]

In summary, cataract development and progression are known as frequent complications of PPV. Because of the application of vitreoretinal surgical techniques to a broader range of posterior segment diseases and because cataract surgery is frequently performed in postvitrectomy eyes, cataract surgeons should be familiar with the challenges of cataract extraction in vitrectomized eyes.

Author details

Olivia Esteban*, Javier Mateo, Paula Casas, Javier Lara and Javier Ascaso
Hospital Clínico Universitario Lozano Blesa, Zaragoza, Spain

*Address all correspondence to: oliviaestebanfloria@hotmail.com

References

[1] Feng H, Adelman RA. Cataract formation following vitreoretinal procedures. Clin Ophthalmol 2014;8:1957-1965.

[2] Panozzo G, Parolini B. Cataracts associated with posterior segment surgery. Opthalmol Clin N Am 2004;17:557-568.

[3] Cherfan GM, Michels RG, de Bustros S, Enger C, Glaser BM. Nuclear sclerotic cataract after vitrectomy for idiopathic epiretinal membranes causing macular pucker. Am J Opthahlmol 1991;111:434-438.

[4] Jackson TL, Nicod E, Angelis A, Grimaccia F, Prevost AT, Simpson ARH, Kanavos P. Pars plana vitrectomy for vitreomacular traction syndrome: a systematic review and metaanalysis of safety and efficacy. Retina. 2013;33:2012-2017.

[5] Jackson TL, Donachie PH, Sparrow JM, Johnston RL. United Kingdom National Ophthalmology Database study of vitreoretinal surgery: report 2, macular hole. Ophthalmology 2013;120:629-634.

[6] Yee KMP, Tan S, Oberstein SYL, Filas B, Nguyen JH, Nguyen-Cuu J, Sebag J. Incidence of cataract surgery after vitrectomy for vitreous opacities. Ophthalmology Retina 2017;1:154-157.

[7] Chang MA, Parides MK, Chang S, Braunstein RE. Outcome of phacoemulsification after pars plana vitrectomy. Ophthalmol 2002;109:948-954.

[8] Thompson JT. The role of patient age and intraocular gas use in cataract progression after vitrectomy for macular holes and epiretinal membranes. Am J Ophthalmol 2004;137:250-257.

[9] Biro Z, Kovacs B. Results of cataract surgery in previously vitrectomized eyes. J Cataract Refract Surg 2002;28:1003-1006.

[10] Titiyal JS, Agarwal E, Angmo D, Sharma M, Kumar A. Comparative evaluation of outcomes of phacoemulsification in vitrectomized eyes: silicone oil versus air/gas group. Int Ophthalmol 2017;37:565-574.

[11] Ahfat FG, Yuen CH, Groenewald CP. Phacoemulsification and intraocular lens implantation following pars plana vitretomy: a prospective eye study. Eye 2003;17:16-20.

[12] Blodi BA, Paluska SA. Cataract after vitrectomy in Young patients. Ophthalmology 1997;104:1092-1095.

[13] Cherfan GM, Michels RG, de Bustros S, Enger C, Glaser BM. Nuclear sclerotic cataract after vitrectomy for idiopathic epiretinal membranes causing macular pucker. Am J Ophthalmol 1991;111:434-438.

[14] Melberg NS, Thomas MA. Nuclear sclerotic cataract after vitrectomy in patients younger than 50 years of age. Ophthalmology 1995;102:1466-1471.

[15] De Bustros S, Thompson JT, Michels RG, Enger C, Rice TA, Glaser BM. Nuclear sclerosis after vitrectomy for idiopathic epiretinal membranes. Am J Ophthalmol 1988;105:160-164.

[16] Truscott RJ. Age-related nuclear cataract-oxidation is the key. Exp Eye Res 2005;80:709-725.

[17] Holekamp NM, Shui YB, Beebe DC. Vitrectomy surgery increases oxygen exposure to the lens: a possible mechanism for nuclear cataract formation. Am J Ophthalmol 2005;139:302-310.

[18] Holekamp NM, Shui YB, Beebe D. Lower intraocular oxygen tension in diabetic patients: possible contribution to decreased incidence of nuclear sclerotic cataract. Am J Ophthalmol 2006;141:1027-1032.

[19] Holekamp NM, Bai F, Shui YB, Almony A, Beebe DC. Ischemic diabetic retinopathy may protect against nuclear sclerotic cataract. Am J Ophthalmol 2010;150:543-550.

[20] Elhousseini Z, Lee E, Williamson TH. Incidence of lens touch during pars plana vitrectomy and outcomes from subsequent cataract surgery. Retina 2016;36:825-829.

[21] Saito Y, Lewis JM, Park I, Ikuno Y, Hayashi A, Ohji M, Tano Y. Nonvitrectomizing vitreous surgery: a strategy to prevent postoperative nuclear sclerosis. Ophthalmology 1999;106:1541-1545.

[22] Sawa M, Saito Y, Hayashi A, Kusaka S, Ohji M, Tano Y. Assessment of nuclear sclerosis after nonvitrectomizing vitreous surgery. Am J Ophthalmol 2001;132:356-362.

[23] Ibarra MS, Hermel M, Prenner JL, Hassan Ts. Longer-term outcomes of transconjuntival sutureless 25-gauge vitrectomy. Am J Ophthalmol 2005;139:831-836.

[24] Faia LJ, McCannel CA, Pulido JS, Hatfield RM, Hatfield ME, McNulty VEW. Outcomes following 25-gauge vitrectomy. Eye 2008;22:1024-1028.

[25] Almony A, Holekamp NM, Bai F, Shui YB, Beebe D. Small-gauge vitrectomy does not protect against nuclear sclerotic cataract. Retina 2012;32:499-505.

[26] Thomas L Lamson 1, Jane Song 2, Azin Abazari 2, Sarah B Weissbart 2. Refractive outcomes of phacoemulsification after pars plana vitrectomy using traditional and new intraocular lens calculation formulas. J Cataract Refract Surg. 2019 Mar;45(3):293-297.

[27] www.zeiss.com/iolmaster700

[28] Vounotrypidis E, Haralanova V, Muth DR, Wertheimer C, Shajari M, Wolf A, Priglinger S, Mayer WJ. Accuracy of SS-OCT biometry compared with partial coherence interferometry biometry for combined phacovitrectomy with internal limiting membrane peeling. J Cataract Refract Surg. 2019 Jan;45(1):48-53.

[29] Shioya M, Ogino N, Shinjo U (1997) Change in postoperative refractive error when vitrectomy is added to intraocular lens implantation. J Cataract Refract Surg 23:1217-1220.

[30] Wang JK, Chang SW. Refractive results of phacoemulsification in vitrectomized patients.Int Ophthalmol. 2017 Jun;37(3):673-681.

[31] Hoffer KJ. Axial length: laser interferometry. Basics of the IOL master. In: Hoffer Kennneth J, editor. Iol power. Thorofare: SLACK; 2011. 63-65.

[32] Mohamed Abou Shousha , Sonia H Yoo. Cataract surgery after pars plana vitrectomy. Curr Opin Ophthalmol. 2010 Jan;21(1):45-49.

[33] Michele Coppola , Alessandro Rabiolo , Maria Vittoria Cicinelli, Giuseppe Querques 2, Francesco Bandello 2. Vitrectomy in high myopia: a narrative review. Int J Retina Vitreous. 2017 Oct 2;3:37.

[34] Yong-Kyu Kim , Se Joon Woo , Joon Young Hyon , Jeeyun Ahn , Kyu Hyung Park . Refractive outcomes of combined phacovitrectomy and delayed cataract surgery in retinal detachment. Can J Ophthalmol. 2015 Oct;50(5):360-366.

[35] Kunavisarut P, Poopattanakul P, Intarated C, Pathanapitoon K. Accuracy and reliability of IOL master and A-scan immersion biometry in silicone oil-filled eyes. Eye (Lond) 2012;26(10):1344-1348.

[36] Roessler GF, Huth JK, Dietlein TS, et al. Accuracy and reproducibilty of axial length measurement in eyes with silicone oil endotemponade. Br J Ophthalmol 2009;93:1492e4.

[37] Piotr Kanclerz 1, Andrzej Grzybowski 2 3. Accuracy of Intraocular Lens Power Calculation in Eyes Filled with Silicone Oil. Semin Ophthalmol. 2019;34(5):392-397.

[38] Hirnschall N, Murphy S, Pimenides D, Maurino V, Findl O. Assessment of a new averaging algorithm to increase the sensitivity of axial eye length measurement with optical biometry in eyes with dense cataract. J Cataract Refract Surg. 2011;37(1):45-49.

[39] Mana Tehrani 1, Frank Krummenauer, Eric Blom, H Burkhard Dick. Evaluation of the practicality of optical biometry and applanation ultrasound in 253 eyes. J Cataract Refract Surg . 2003 Apr;29(4):741-746.

[40] Piotr Kanclerz 1, Andrzej Grzybowski 2 3. Accuracy of Intraocular Lens Power Calculation in Eyes Filled with Silicone Oil. Semin Ophthalmol. 2019;34(5):392-397.

[41] Hoffer KJ. Special circumstances silicone oil power. In: Hoffer Kennneth J, editor. Iol power. Thorofare: SLACK; 2011. 221-222

[42] Hoffer KJ. Ultrasound velocities for axial eye length measurement. J Cataract Refract Surg 1994;20:554-562.

[43] Khaled G Abu El Einen 1, Mervat H Shalaby, Hoda T El Shiwy.Immersion B-guided versus contact A-mode biometry for accurate measurement of axial length and intraocular lens power calculation in siliconized eyes. Retina. 2011 Feb;31(2):262-265.

[44] Silicone OiL Retinal Detachments IOL Power Calculations. East Valley Ophthalmology. http://www.doctor-hill.com/iol-main/silicone.htm.

[45] M A Rehman Siddiqui 1, M Amer Awan, Andrew Fairhead, Hatem Atta. Ultrasound velocity in heavy ocular tamponade agents and implications for biometry. Br J Ophthalmol . 2011 Jan;95(1):142-144.

[46] Murray DC, Potamitis T, Good P, et al. Biometry of the silicone oil-filled eye. Eye 1999;13:319-324.

[47] Takei K, Sekine Y, Okamoto F, Hommura S. Measurement of axial length of eyes with incomplete filling of silicone oil in the vitreous cavity using x ray computed tomography. Br J Ophthalmol. 2002;86(1):47-50.

[48] Zaldivar R, Shultz MC, Davidorf JM, Holladay JT. Intraocular lens power calculations in patients with extreme myopia. J Cataract Refract Surg 2000; 26:668-674.

[49] Hammouda Hamdi Ghoraba 1, Alaa Amer El-Dorghamy, Ahmed Fahmy Atia, Abd El-Aziz Ismail Yassin. The problems of biometry in combined silicone oil removal and cataract extraction: a clinical trial. Retina. 2002 Oct;22(5):589-596.

[50] Larkin GB, Flaxel CJ, Leaver PK. Phacoemulsification and silicone oil removal through a single corneal incision. Ophthalmologe 1998;105: 2023-2027.

[51] Assi A, Woodruff S, Gotzaridis E, Bunce C, Sullivan P. Combined phacoemulsification and transpupillary drainage of silicone

oil: results and complications. Br J Ophthalmol 2001; 85:942-945.

[52] Nawrocki J, Ghoraba H, Gabel VP. Problems with silicon oil removal. A study of 63 consecutive cases. Ophthalmologe 1993;90:258-263.

[53] Grinbaum A, Treister G, Moisseiev J. Predicted and actual refraction after intraocular lens implantation in eyes with silicone oil. J Cataract Refract Surg 1996;22:726-729.

[54] Shira Sheen Ophir, Asaf Friehmann, Alexander Rubowitz. Circumferential silicone sponge scleral buckling induced axial length changes: case series and comparison to literature. Int J Retina Vitreous. 2017 Mar 27;3:10.

[55] Lee DH, Han JW, Kim SS, Byeon SH, Koh HJ, Lee SC, Kim M. Long-term Effect of Scleral Encircling on Axial Elongation. Am J Ophthalmol. 2018 May;189:139-145.

[56] Batman C, Cekic O. Phacoemulsification and silicone oil removal through a single incision. Ophthalmologe 1999;106:1234-1236.

[57] V G Madanagopalan 1, Pradeep Susvar 1, M Arthi 2. Refractive outcomes of a single-step and a two-step approach for silicone oil removal and cataract surgery. Indian J Ophthalmol . 2019 May;67(5):625-629.

[58] Samir Mohamed El-Baha 1, Tarek Samir Hemeida Comparison of refractive outcome using intraoperative biometry and partial coherence interferometry in silicone oil-filled eyes. Retina. 2009 Jan;29(1):64-68.

[59] Amal M Elbendary 1, Mohamed M Elwan.Predicted versus actual intraocular lens power in silicon-oil-filled eyes undergoing cataract extraction using automated intraoperative retinoscopy. Curr Eye Res. 2012 Aug;37(8):694-697.

[60] Hill W. Understanding silicone oil. Mesa Arizona. [cited 2020 November 1]; Available in: https://doctor-hill.com/iol-power-calculations/silicone-oil/.

[61] Joris Vander Mijnsbrugge 1, Jean-Francois Fils 2, Joyce Jansen 3, Minh-Tri Hua 3, Peter Stalmans 3. The role of the vitreous body in effective IOL positioning. Graefes Arch Clin Exp Ophthalmol. 2018 Aug;256(8):1517-1520.

[62] Gülkilik G, Erdur S, Özbek M, Özsütcü M, Adabasi M, Demirci G, Kocabora M, Eliacik M (2016) Changes in anterior chamber depth after combined phacovitrectomy. Turk J Ophthalmol 46:161-164

[63] Meira Neudorfer 1, Nir Oren, Adiel Barak. High-frequency ultrasound biomicroscopy of the anterior segment morphometry before and immediately after pars plana vitrectomy. Eur J Ophthalmol . Mar-Apr 2011;21(2):173-178

[64] Li Y, Yang CX, Qing GP,WeiWB (2013) Changes in anterior chamber depth following vitrectomy. Chin Med J 126(19):3701-3704

[65] Hamoudi H, La Cour M.Refractive changes after vitrectomy and phacovitrectomy for macular hole and epiretinal membrane. J Cataract Refract Surg.2013;39:942-947.

[66] Chunmei Huang 1, Tonghe Zhang 1, Jian Liu 1, Qiang Ji 2, Ruili Tan 1. Changes in axial length, central cornea thickness, and anterior chamber depth after rhegmatogenous retinal detachment repair. BMC Ophthalmol. 2016 Jul 25;16:121.

[67] Nobuhiko Shiraki , Taku Wakabayashi , Hirokazu Sakaguchi , Kohji Nishida . Effect of Gas Tamponade on the Intraocular Lens Position and Refractive Error after Phacovitrectomy: A Swept-Source Anterior Segment

OCT Analysis. Ophthalmology . 2020 Apr;127(4):511-515.

[68] Na Young Lee , Shin Hae Park, Choun Ki Joo. Refractive outcomes of phacoemulsification and intraocular lens implantation after pars plana vitrectomy. Retina. 2009 Apr;29(4):487-491.

[69] Tan X, Zhang J, Zhu Y, Xu J, Qiu X, Yang G, Liu Z, Luo L, Liu Y. Accuracy of New Generation Intraocular Lens Calculation Formulas in Vitrectomized Eyes. Am J Ophthalmol. 2020 Sep;217:81-90.

[70] Paris G Tranos, Bruce Allan , Miltiadis Balidis , Athanasios Vakalis, Solon Asteriades , George Anogeianakis, Magda Triantafilla, Nikolaos Kozeis, Panagiotis Stavrakas. Comparison of postoperative refractive outcome in eyes undergoing combined phacovitrectomy vs cataract surgery following vitrectomy. Graefes Arch Clin Exp Ophthalmol. 2020 May;258(5):987-993.

[71] Nobuhiko Shiraki , Taku Wakabayashi , Hirokazu Sakaguchi, Kohji Nishida . Optical Biometry-Based Intraocular Lens Calculation and Refractive Outcomes after Phacovitrectomy for Rhegmatogenous Retinal Detachment and Epiretinal Membrane. Sci Rep. 2018 Jul 27;8(1):11319..

[72] Kelly D Schweitzer , Raúl García.Myopic shift after combined phacoemulsification and vitrectomy with gas tamponade. Can J Ophthalmol. 2008 Oct;43(5):581-583.

[73] Leonie J van der Geest , Martin J Siemerink 1, Marco Mura , Maarten P Mourits , Ruth Lapid-Gortzak 2.Refractive outcomes after phacovitrectomy surgery. J Cataract Refract Surg. 2016 Jun;42(6):840-845.

[74] Misra A, Burton RL. Incidence of intraoperative complications during phacoemulsification in vitrectomized and nonvitrectomized eyes: prospective study. J Cataract Refract Surg. 2005 May;31(5):1011-1014.

[75] Biro Z, Kovacs B. Results of cataract surgery in previously vitrectomized eyes. J Cataract Refract Surg 2002; 28: 1003-1006.

[76] Chang MA, Parides MK, Chang S, Braunstein RE. Out- come of phacoemulsification after pars plana vitrectomy. Ophthalmology 2002; 109:948-954.

[77] Lacalle VD, Ga´rate FJO, Alday NM, et al. Phacoemulsi- fication cataract surgery in vitrectomized eyes. J Cataract Refract Surg 1998; 24:806-809.

[78] Biro Z, Kovacs B. Results of cataract surgery in previously vitrectomized eyes. J Cataract Refract Surg 2002; 28: 1003-1006.

[79] Misra A, Burton RL. Incidence of intraoperative complications during phacoemulsification in vitrectomized and nonvitrectomized eyes: prospective study. J Cataract Refract Surg. 2005 May;31(5):1011-1014.

[80] Braunstein RE, Airiani S. Cataract surgery results after pars plana vitrectomy. Curr Opin Ophthalmol 2003; 14:150-154.

[81] Sachdev N, Brar GS, Sukhija J, et al. Phacoemulsification in vitrectomized eyes: results using a 'phaco chop' technique. Acta Ophthalmol. 2009;87(4): 382-385.

[82] Ghosh S, Best K, Steel DH. Lens-iris diaphragm retropulsion syndrome during phacoemulsification in vitrectomized eyes. J Cataract Refract Surg. 2013;39(12):1852-1858.

[83] Titiyal JS, Agarwal E, Angmo D, et al. Comparative evaluation of outcomes of phacoemulsification in

vitrectomized eyes: silicone oil versus air/gas group. Int Ophthalmol 2016.

[84] Gimbel HV, DeBroff BM. Intraocular lens optic capture. J Cataract Refract Surg. 2004 Jan;30(1):200-206.

[85] Rey A, Jürgens I, Maseras X, Dyrda A, Pera P, Morilla A. Visual outcome and complications of cataract extraction after pars plana vitrectomy. Clin Ophthalmol. 2018 May 25;12:989-994.

[86] Titiyal JS, Agarwal E, Angmo D, Sharma N, Kumar A. Comparative evaluation of outcomes of phacoemulsification in vitrectomized eyes: silicone oil versus air/gas group. Int Ophthalmol. 2017;37(3):565-574.

[87] Ahfat FG, Yuen CH, Groenewald CP. Phacoemulsification and intraocular lens implantation following pars plana vitretomy: a prospective eye study. Eye. 2003;17(1):16-20.

[88] Ahfat FG, Yuen CH, Groenewald CP. Phacoemulsification and intraocular lens implantation following pars plana vitrectomy: a prospective study. Eye 2003; 17: 16-20.

[89] Chang MA, Parides MK, Chang S et al. Outcome of phacoemulsification after pars plana vitrectomy. Ophthalmology 2002; 109: 948-954.

[90] Biro Z, Kovacs B. Results of cataract surgery in previously vitrectomized eyes. J Cataract Refract Surg 2002; 28: 1003-1006.

[91] Chang MA, Parides MK, Chang S, Braunstein RE. Outcome of phacoemulsification after pars plana vitrectomy. Ophthalmology. 2002; 109(5):948-954.

[92] Shaumberg DA, Dana MR, Christen WG, Glynn RJ. Asystematicover- view of the incidence of posterior capsule opacification. Ophthalmology. 1998; 105(7):1213-1221.

[93] Rey A, Jürgens I, Dyrda A, et al. Surgical outcome of late in-the-bag intraocular lens dislocation treated with pars plana vitrectomy. Retina 2016;36(3):576-581.

Chapter 4

Special Cases in Cataract Surgery

Minghui Deng, Song Chen and Xiaogang Wang

Abstract

During phacoemulsification for cataracts, the surgeon may encounter various challenges and should therefore be trained to handle them. This chapter will share an example of clinical cases encountered by the author in clinical practice, which mainly includes the successful implantation of a trifocal intraocular lens in the capsular bag after posterior capsular tear during posterior polar cataract surgery as well as cataract surgery design after corneal refractive surgery, shrinkage, and treatment of capsular opening in patients with retinitis pigmentosa after cataract surgery to provide a reference for clinicians.

Keywords: posterior polar cataract, retinitis pigmentosa, post-corneal refractive surgery, phacoemulsification surgery for cataract

1. Introduction

With continuous advancements in technology, emergence of new equipment, and introduction of new types of intraocular lens (IOL) for cataract surgery, the latter has entered the era of refractive surgery. Simultaneously, the advent of a variety of functional IOLs [1] can enable patients to achieve functional vision recovery after cataract surgery. The individualized eye conditions of the patient and the unpredictable special conditions that occur during and after surgery should be considered by every cataract surgeon. Based on our clinical experience, the following are a few questions for readers to contemplate: (1) After the occurrence of posterior capsule circular capsulorhexis and posterior capsular rupture, can high-end IOLs be safely implanted? (2) For cataract patients with obvious decentered ablation after laser-assisted in-situ keratomileusis (LASIK), is high-end IOL implantation suitable during phacoemulsification? (3) How can we deal with capsular shrinkage syndrome after cataract surgery in patients with retinitis pigmentosa and high myopia?

In the following chapters, we will specifically report the three aforementioned situations in combination with actual cases, for providing readers with valuable clinical references.

2. A case of successful implantation of a trifocal intraocular lens in the capsular bag after posterior capsule tear in posterior polar cataract surgery

A 25-year-old male patient was admitted to the hospital for a complaint of blurred vision in the right eye since childhood, which had gradually aggravated and was accompanied by photophobia for 2 years. The patient had refractive errors bilaterally and amblyopia in his right eye and had worn glasses for many years.

The eye examination revealed that the right eye had a visual acuity of 0.25, which could not be corrected; the left eye had a visual acuity of 0.1, wherein optometry showed (−2.50 D), and it was corrected to 1.0; the binocular intraocular pressure was normal. The right eye lens was disc-shaped, irregular porcelain, with white opacity seen in the posterior pole, and the left eye lens was transparent (**Figure 1**). The corneal endothelial cell count of the right eye was 2479.9 cells/mm^2; No abnormality was evident in the optical coherence tomography (OCT) examination of the macular area. His condition was diagnosed as a posterior polar cataract of the right eye, amblyopia in the right eye, and refractive error in the left eye.

The patient was only 25 years old and had certain requirements for a full range of vision; however, the right eye of the patient had a posterior polar cataract. Based on the results of Pentacam, the posterior capsule was very likely to be severely organized or incomplete, and the patient had amblyopia in the right eye. Therefore, before the operation, the patient was informed about the surgical procedure such that the patient fully understood that the posterior capsule might be organized, opaque, or incomplete during the operation, and it would be necessary to perform posterior capsule continuous circular capsulorhexis. If the capsulorhexis was successful, then a trifocal IOL could be implanted. Otherwise, a prepared three-piece single-focus IOL would be implanted. Even if the trifocal IOL was successfully implanted, the postoperative far, medium, and near visions would not reach the normal level due to amblyopia and would need to be corrected by wearing glasses. With the patient's full understanding, the right eye cataract phacoemulsification and trifocal IOL implantation was performed on March 31, 2020. Before the

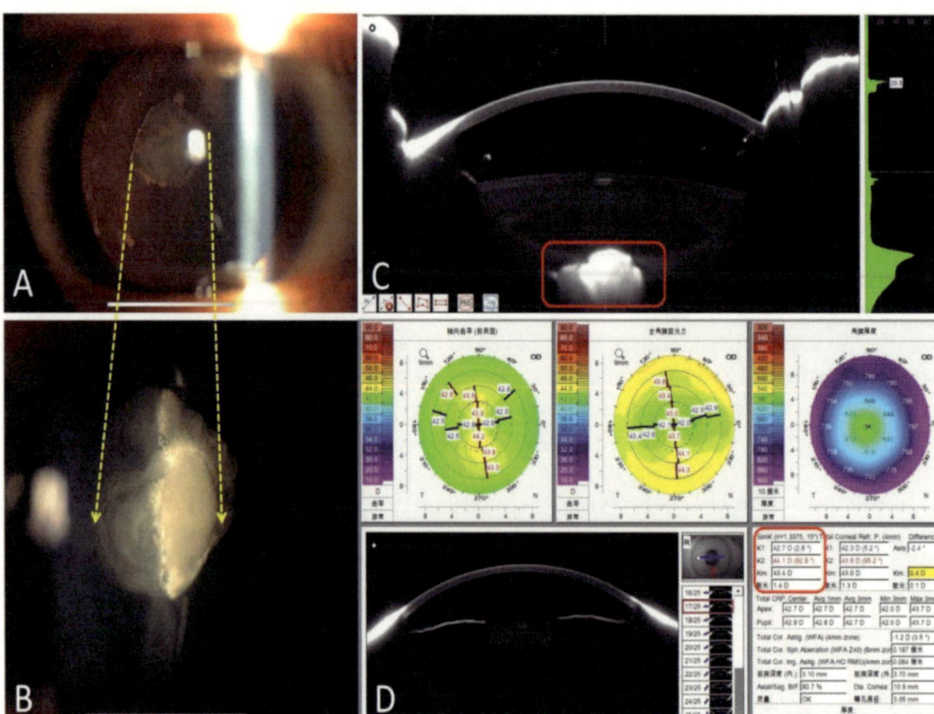

Figure 1.
Slit-lamp photography after mydriasis of the surgical eye shows that the posterior capsule is opaque, dense, and organized (A, B). Pentacam examination after mydriasis shows that the posterior capsule is opaque and demonstrates high reflective brightness, with a high brightness value (C red box); there is 1.4 D@93° regular corneal astigmatism at 15° of the center of the anterior surface of the cornea under the measurement of the natural pupil (D red box).

operation, the 0-180° axial position was marked in the surgical eye in the sitting position. After routine disinfection and draping during the operation, the Placido disc marked the meridian position of the steep axis of corneal astigmatism at the 93° and 273° axial positions of the surgical eye; a 3.0-mm skeratome was then used to make a symmetric incision at the corneal limbus of the steep axis of the cornea, and 5.5-mm continuous circular capsulorhexis and hydrodelineation were performed. Phacoemulsification was used to aspirate and remove the nucleus and cortex. The posterior capsule was not found to be incomplete; however, the thick white mass of the opaque, organized tissue attached to the upper center of the posterior capsule could not be polished or aspirated. The viscoelastic agent was injected into the anterior chamber, and a 1-mL syringe needle was used to remove the opaque, organized tissue that adhered to the posterior capsule. Subsequently, a posterior capsule continuous circular capsulorhexis of approximately 4.0 mm was successfully performed, and while a +19.0 D trifocal IOL (AT LISA tri 839mp, Zeiss) was implanted in the capsular bag, during which the IOL was rapidly unfolded. It was found that the posterior capsule annular capsulorhexis opening had partial dehiscence at approximately the 8 o' clock position; however, no vitreous was observed. The IOL was rotated to make its long axis perpendicular to the angle of the posterior capsule dehiscence such that the IOL was centered in the capsular bag, the residual viscoelastic agent in the anterior chamber was aspirated, and the stability and centering of the IOL were verified again. The incision was watertight and the IOL position was observed to ensure that it was centered, and the operation was complete (**Figure 2**).

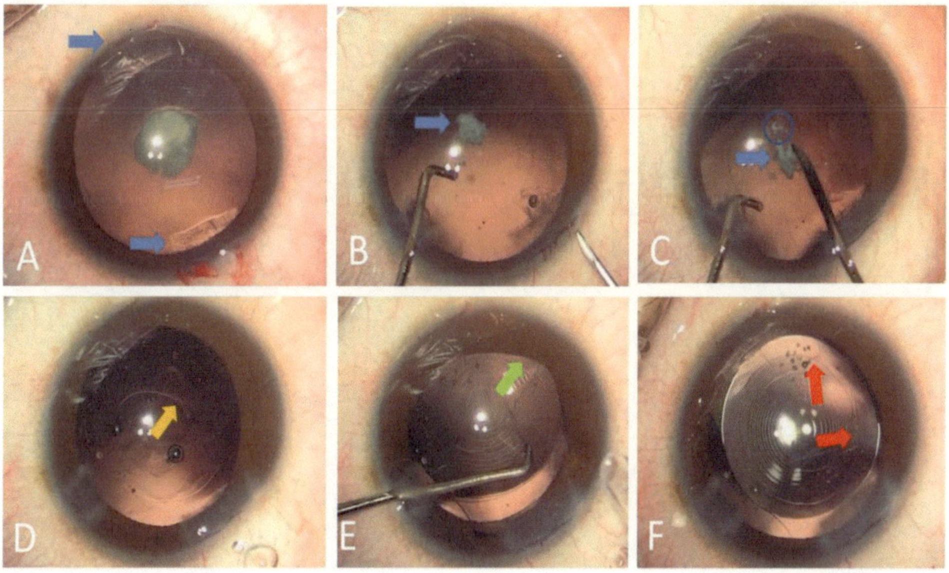

Figure 2.
According to the preoperative corneal astigmatism of the patient, a 3.0-mm-wide symmetric transparent corneal incision was made on the steep axis of the cornea to relieve corneal astigmatism (A, blue arrow). After the nucleus and cortex were aspirated, the thick white mass of opaque and organized tissue attached to the upper center of the posterior capsule could not be polished or aspirated (B, blue arrow). A 1-mL syringe needle was used to remove the opaque and organized tissues that adhered to the posterior capsule (C, blue arrow and the blue circular area). After the completion of the continuous circular capsulorhexis of the posterior capsule, there were manifestations of the irregular capsulorhexis opening at nearly the 8 o' clock position, which was a hidden danger for the subsequent occurrence of posterior capsular rupture at this location (D, yellow arrow); the plate-type trifocal intraocular lens (IOL) was rapidly unfolded during implantation, and pressure was applied to the weak part at nearly the 8 o' clock position of the posterior capsular opening to cause rupture (E, green arrow); finally, the long axis of the IOL was placed in the direction perpendicular to the posterior capsular dehiscence angle, the IOL was stable and centered, and, simultaneously, the dehiscence site of the posterior capsulorhexis opening and the opaque and organized site in Figure D corresponded to each other (F, red arrow).

The uncorrected visual acuity of the right eye was (far vision 0.4, medium vision 0.4 near vision 0.63) at 1 day after operation, (far vision 0.5, medium vision 0.5, near vision 0.63) at 1 week after operation, and (far vision 0.5, medium vision 0.5, near vision 0.63) at 42 days after operation, and (far vision 0.5, medium vision 0.5, near vision 0.63), optometry showing −0.75DCX138°, which was corrected to +0.5 at 7 months after operation. At this time, the IOL position was stable and centered as revealed in reexamination (**Figure 3**). There were no manifestations of anisometropia or complaints of obvious glare, halo, and other adverse visual phenomena in the postoperative reexaminations at various stages.

2.1 Discussion

In this study, a patient with amblyopia and a monocular posterior polar cataract in the right eye was analyzed. The with-the-rule corneal astigmatism (around 1.4D) was partially corrected by using a steep-axis clear corneal symmetric incision during the operation. Considering the potential influence of the densely opaque and organized tissue in the visual axis of posterior capsule, a posterior capsule continuous circular capsulorhexis was successfully performed during the surgery, and a trifocal IOL was implanted in the capsular bag. However, when the trifocal IOL was implanted as the hydrophilic acrylic IOL was unfolded rapidly, it caused pressure

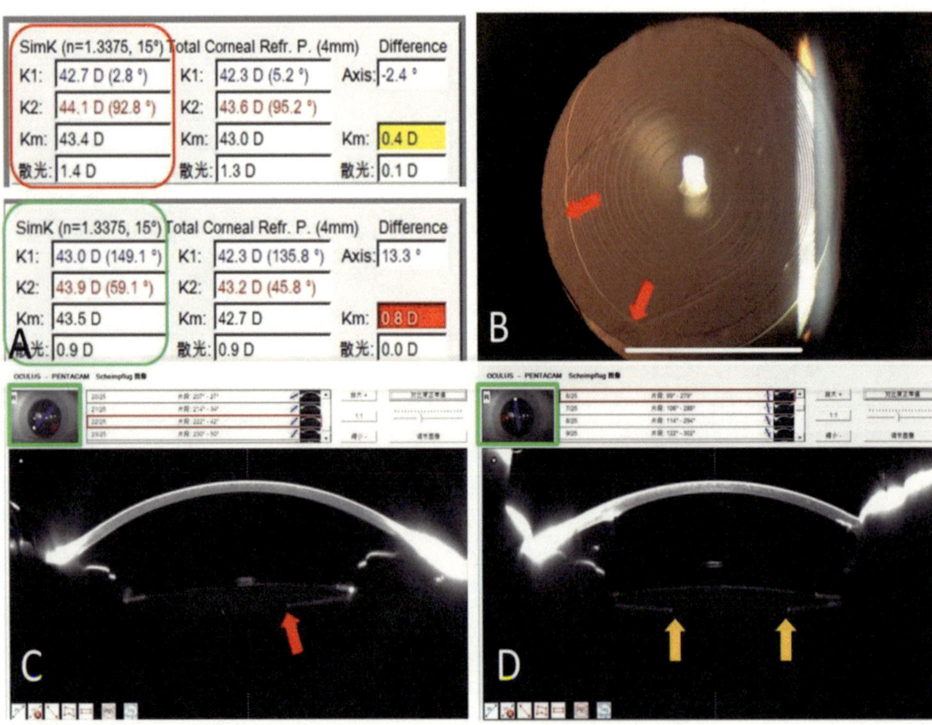

Figure 3.
Pentacam examination performed again at 7 months after surgery shows that the anterior surface corneal astigmatism changed from 1.4 D@93° before surgery to 0.9 D@59° (A, red frame and green frame); Slit-lamp retroillumination imaging showing that the intraocular lens was centered and stable, the dehiscence of the posterior capsular opening at the 8 o' clock position did not change significantly compared to the intraoperative status (B, red arrow); Pentacam tomography showing that the posterior capsule signal at the 8 o' clock position is discontinuous and no contralateral signal is observed, indicating the direction of posterior capsule dehiscence (C, green box and red arrow); Pentacam tomography scan showing that the posterior capsule is incomplete in the direction of nearly the 6 o' clock position; however, the signal of the margin of the posterior capsule is visible and symmetrical (D, green box and yellow arrow).

on the weak posterior capsule circular capsulorhexis opening, and the dehiscence of posterior capsulorhexis opening occurred. As the posterior capsule and anterior hyaloid membrane were separated with a viscoelastic agent in advance, there was no vitreous overflow. By rotating the position of the IOL, the long axis of the IOL was perpendicular to the direction of the dehiscence of posterior capsulorhexis opening and the four corner loops of the plate-type IOL provided support in the capsular bag, thus ensuring its centering and stability. Although the patient had amblyopia and large astigmatism in the surgical eye, he received full explaination before the operation to ensure his recognition and understanding. The postoperative corneal astigmatism was controlled within 1.0 D, and the far, medium, and near visions were greatly improved compared to those before the operation; the postoperative patient satisfaction was quite high. In 2018, Srinivasaraghavan et al. reported a case of successful implantation of a functional IOL in the capsular bag after a posterior capsule rupture in a traumatic cataract patient, which provided a certain reference basis for this study [2].

The choice of the trifocal IOL for this case is mainly based on the following considerations: (1) Young patients have a high demand for a full range of vision; (2) Although the patient's cornea had 1.4 D with-the-rule astigmatism, studies have shown that after the production of a symmetric transparent corneal incision on the steep axis of the cornea, a 2.8–3.5 mm clear corneal incision could correct 1.00-2.06 D of astigmatism [3–5]. Based on the surgeon's previous surgical experience, it was considered that astigmatism could be reduced to less than 1.0 D through the symmetric incision on the steep axis of the cornea. Simultaneously, according to the correction analysis of the astigmatism IOL using the Baylor nomogram, it was not necessary to correct with-the-rule astigmatism of less than 1.69 D, which also provided the basis for the implantation of the trifocal IOL in this study [6]; (3) Except for the posterior polar cataract, no organic abnormality was evident in the patient's surgical eye examination. However, through a retrospective analysis of the patient's medical history and various examinations, he was diagnosed as amblyopia, and it was expected that although the postoperative visual acuity could not reach normal, it would be greatly improved compared with the preoperative visual acuity, and the full range of visual acuity could be achieved; therefore, the final choice was to implant a trifocal IOL.

Posterior polar cataract surgery is highly challenging and unpredictable, because the specific conditions of the posterior capsule must always be considered during the operation; only hydrodelineation, without hydrodissection, is performed during the operation, and the anterior chamber must be maintained stable at all times to avoid causing excessive tension on the posterior capsule and thus resulting in posterior capsule rupture [7–9]. Although the posterior capsule of this patient was intact during the operation, its opacity was located in the visual axis, which seriously affected the visual quality after IOL implantation. Therefore, the posterior capsule was subjected to continuous circular capsulorhexis during the operation [9]. When a trifocal IOL was implanted, it was unfolded quickly and caused great tension on the posterior capsulorhexis opening, leading to dehiscence of the posterior capsulorhexis opening. The location of the dehiscence of the posterior capsular was the same as the site where the capsulorhexis crossed over the opacity of the posterior capsule. Considering that the tension resistance of the capsule here was weaker than that of the normal posterior capsule, dehiscence occurred under the state of uneven tension when the IOL was unfolded after implantation. This also suggests that we should try to tear off the opacity part as far as possible during the posterior capsule capsulorhexis to ensure even and consistent tension resistance of the capsular opening.

After the intraoperative implantation of a trifocal IOL, the dehiscence of posterior capsulorhexis opening occurred beyond our expectation. We must weigh the pros and cons according to the specific situation. If the trifocal IOL could not be stably implanted in the capsular bag or if there was a large amount of vitreous overflow, then we would choose to implant a single focal three-piece IOL in the ciliary sulcus, and the optical part was captured in the anterior capsulorhexis opening of less than 6 mm, which could prevent the eccentricity and tilt of the IOL that might occur after surgery and keep its stability [10]. The surgeon assessed that although the posterior capsular capsulorhexis dehiscence occurred during the intraoperative trifocal IOL implantation in this patient, the anterior vitreous membrane was well protected in the early stage and there was no vitreous overflow; therefore, the long axis of trifocal IOL was rotated to the direction perpendicular to the direction of dehiscence, which reduced further pulling of the IOL on the capsulorhexis opening of dehiscence and allowed it to be stable and centered in the capsular bag.

Although this study did not involve a follow-up for 1 year or longer after surgery, the long-term stability of the trifocal IOL remained to be observed; however, this study emphasizes that for posterior capsular continuous circular capsulorhexis in posterior polar cataract surgery or a small range of posterior capsular rupture in common cataract surgery followed by posterior capsular continuous circular capsulorhexis, in circumstances where there is no vitreous overflow, the surgeon can evaluate whether it is feasible to implant the trifocal IOL in the capsular bag according to the actual intraoperative situation and expand the relative indications for trifocal IOL surgery.

3. A case of trifocal intraocular lens implantation for high myopia complicated with cataract after LASIK operation

A 51-year-old male patient underwent LASIK surgery 23 years ago due to high myopia in both eyes. According to the patient's recollection, the best postoperative visual acuity in his eyes was 0.5 in the right eye and 0.6 in the left eye. On May 20, 2019, the patient presented with high myopia and cataract in both eyes, binocular visions: right eye 0.08, left eye 0.12; optometry: right eye −14.50DS = 0.3, left eye −13.50DS/−0.75 DC*50° = 0.3. The fundus photos and OCT scanning of both eyes showed high myopic retinal changes (**Figure 4**).

The corneal topography examination showed obvious decentered ablation (**Figure 5**), and the right eye's total corneal astigmatism was 1.3 D, total corneal spherical aberration (SA) was 0.532 μm, total corneal irregular astigmatism was 1.615 μm, and angle kappa was 0.79 mm. The left eye's total corneal astigmatism was 2.4 D, total corneal SA was 1.259 μm, and total corneal irregular astigmatism was 1.373 μm. The above indicators were significantly beyond the scope of application of the trifocal IOL recommended by the Expert Consensus on The Clinical Application of Multifocal IOLs in China (2019): estimated postoperative total corneal astigmatism $\leq$ 0.75 D, preoperative total corneal spherical aberration (SA) $\leq$ 0.3 μm, total corneal irregular astigmatism $\leq$ 0.3 to 0.5 μm, angle kappa $\leq$ 0.5 mm, or less than half of the diameter of the central refractive optical zone of the IOL.

Given the actual situation of the patient, we conducted in-depth communication with the patient and recommended that the patient should receive an implant of a single-focus IOL to avoid evident symptoms of visual discomfort after the operation. However, the patient had a strong willing of not wearing eyeglasses after surgry; therefore, he still wanted to apply trifocal IOL to achieve full range of vision after surgery. Even in the event of maladaptation, he was willing to replace the IOL with another operation.

Finally, it was decided to perform phacoemulsification combined with trifocal IOL implantation on the right eye, which had relatively good corneal conditions.

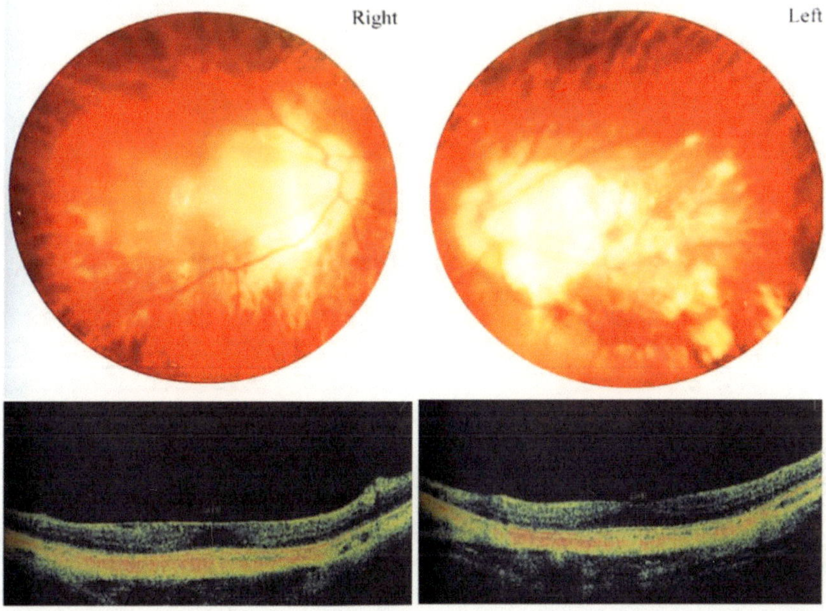

Figure 4.
Fundus photography and OCT examination showing high myopic changes in the fundus of both eyes.

In this case, a multi-formula average method from the American Society of Cataract and Refractive Surgery (ASCRS) website was used for IOL power calculation to improve the accuracy. Because the patient's right eye corneal astigmatism was 1.3D, we used a 3.0-mm symmetrical and clear corneal incision on the 101.9° meridian of the steep axis of the cornea to partially correct the corneal astigmatism. Subsequently, continuous circular capsulorhexis with a diameter of approximately 5.5 mm was performed during the operation, and the phacoemulsification was completed using the Stellaris (Bausch +Lomb Laboratories, USA) system. After aspirating cortex, the anterior and posterior capsules were thoroughly polished, and +10.0 D (IOL degrees of both eyes are selected according to the ASCRS IOL Calculator for Eyes with Prior Myopic LASIK/PRK online calculation formula) Zeiss trifocal IOL (AT LISA tri839MP) was implanted; no complications occurred during the operation.

Visual acuity on the second day of right eye was as follows: far vision 0.4, medium vision 0.63, near vision 0.63; optometry showed that the far vision was −0.5 DS/−0.75 DC*105°=0.5 and intraocular pressure was 15 mmHg; slit-lamp examination showed that the cornea was transparent and clear, and the clear corneal incision was well closed; the pupil was sensitive to light, and the IOL was well-centered (**Figure 6**). The Pentacam examination of the right eye showed that the corneal incision was well closed, and the patient was highly satisfied and did not complain of any visual disturbance or discomfort.

Given the more obvious decentered ablation of the left cornea, greater corneal astigmatism, and greater total corneal SA and total corneal irregular astigmatism (**Figure 5**), we communicated with the patient repeatedly to inform about the possible obvious visual disturbance and discomfort after surgery. After the patient's approval to use the ZEISS trifocal IOL, we used the same method to perform left eye phacoemulsification combined with +9.5 D Zeiss trifocal IOL implantation for the patient on May 28, 2019. There were no complications during the operation.

On May 29, 2019, a re-examination showed that the right eye had a far vision of 0.5, medium vision of 0.63, and near vision of 0.63, and the left eye had a far vision of 0.5, medium vision of 0.5, and near vision of 0.5. Optometry showed that the

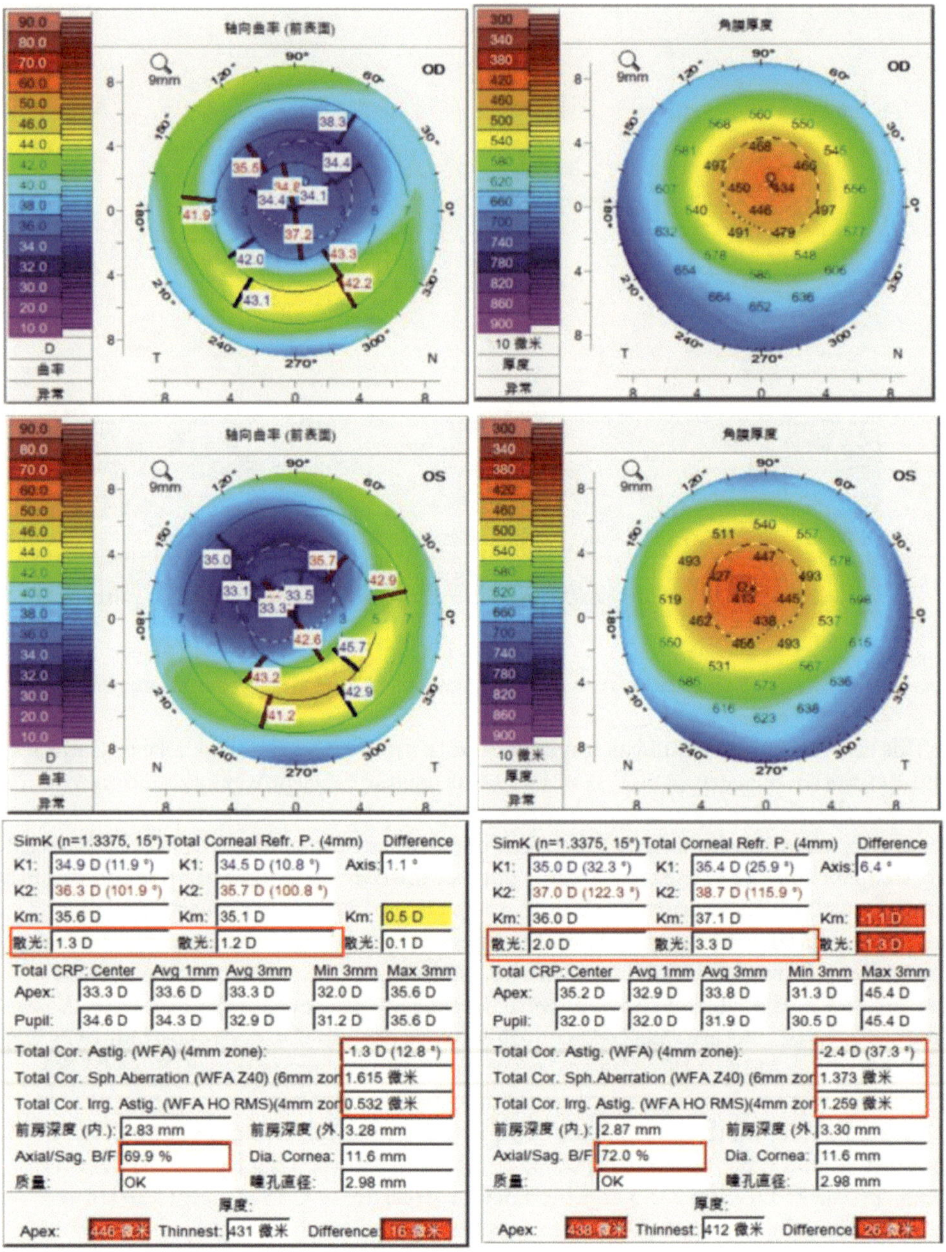

Figure 5.
Binocular Pentacam examination showing decentered ablation in both eyes.

right eye had −0.75 DC*107°=0.5 and the left eye had −0.25 DS/−0.5 DC*135°=0.5. The intraocular pressure was 14 mmHg in the right eye and 16 mmHg in the left eye. Slit-lamp examination showed that the cornea of both eyes was transparent and clear, the clear corneal incision was well closed, the pupils were sensitive to light, and the IOL was well-centered (**Figure 7**). On June 05, 2019, the results of Pentacam examination performed again on both eyes showed that the corneal incision was well closed, the corneal astigmatism in both eyes was reduced compared with that before the operation, and the total corneal SA and total corneal irregular astigmatism were both reduced compared with those before the operation. The patient was highly satisfied, which was a completely unexpected outcome (**Figure 8**).

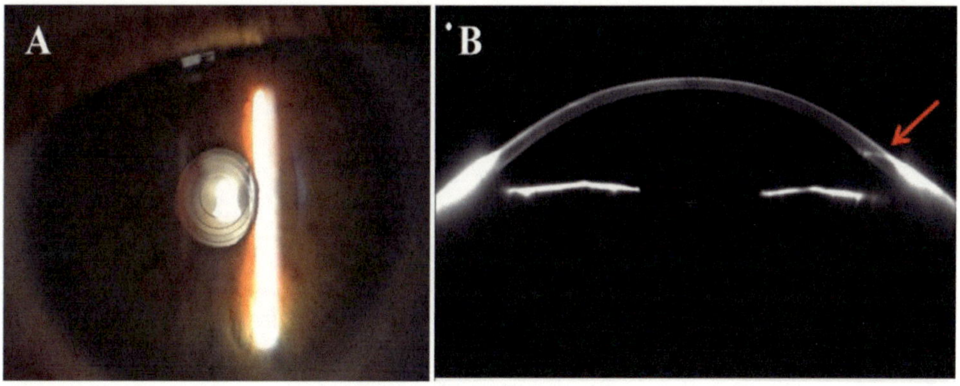

Figure 6.
A right-eye slit-lamp photograph taken on May 24, 2019, showing the trifocal intraocular lens (IOL) is well centered, and the center of the diffraction ring is quite close to the center of the pupil (Panel A). Simultaneously, Pentacam in the right eye shows that the corneal incision is well closed (red arrow in Panel B).

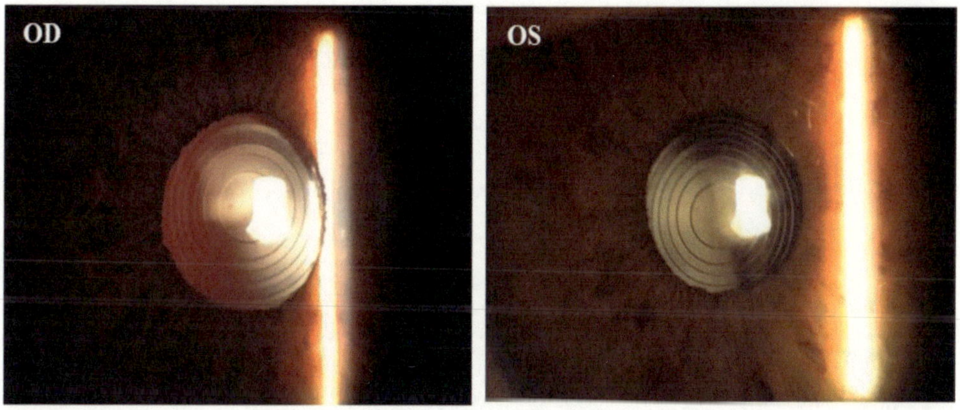

Figure 7.
A binocular slit-lamp photograph taken on May 29, 2019, showing that the trifocal intraocular lens (IOL) is well centered, and the center of the diffraction ring is quite close to the center of the pupil.

3.1 Discussion

Since 1990s, corneal refractive surgery has been widely performed for refractive correction in millions of younger patients. As they grew older for cataract surgery, they are still willing to acquire better visual quality and freedom from glasses [11]. Some of previous studies have demonstrated that multifocal IOL implantation could be a safe and efficient way for patients with previous corneal refractive surgery [12–15]. However, due to the uncertainty in IOL power calculation and the potential side effects such as glare, halo or other visual acuity problems, premium IOL surgical plans for patients post-corneal refractive surgery are still facing many challenges.

AT LISA tri839MP used in this study, as a monolithic diffractive trifocal IOL, is able to split the incoming light at near, intermediate, and distant focus, respectively. It has been shown to provide good outcomes of visual acuity at a near, intermediate, and far distance and a high postoperative satisfaction [16, 17]. Moreover, two previous studies also demonstrated that it can provide a good visual outcome at both near and distance vision for post-myopic LASIK cases [18, 19].

Although the patient's corneal astigmatism, irregular astigmatism, and SA in both eyes exceeded the scope of application of the Zeiss trifocal IOL, the patient had a strong willingness of not wearing eyeglasses after the operation. Therefore,

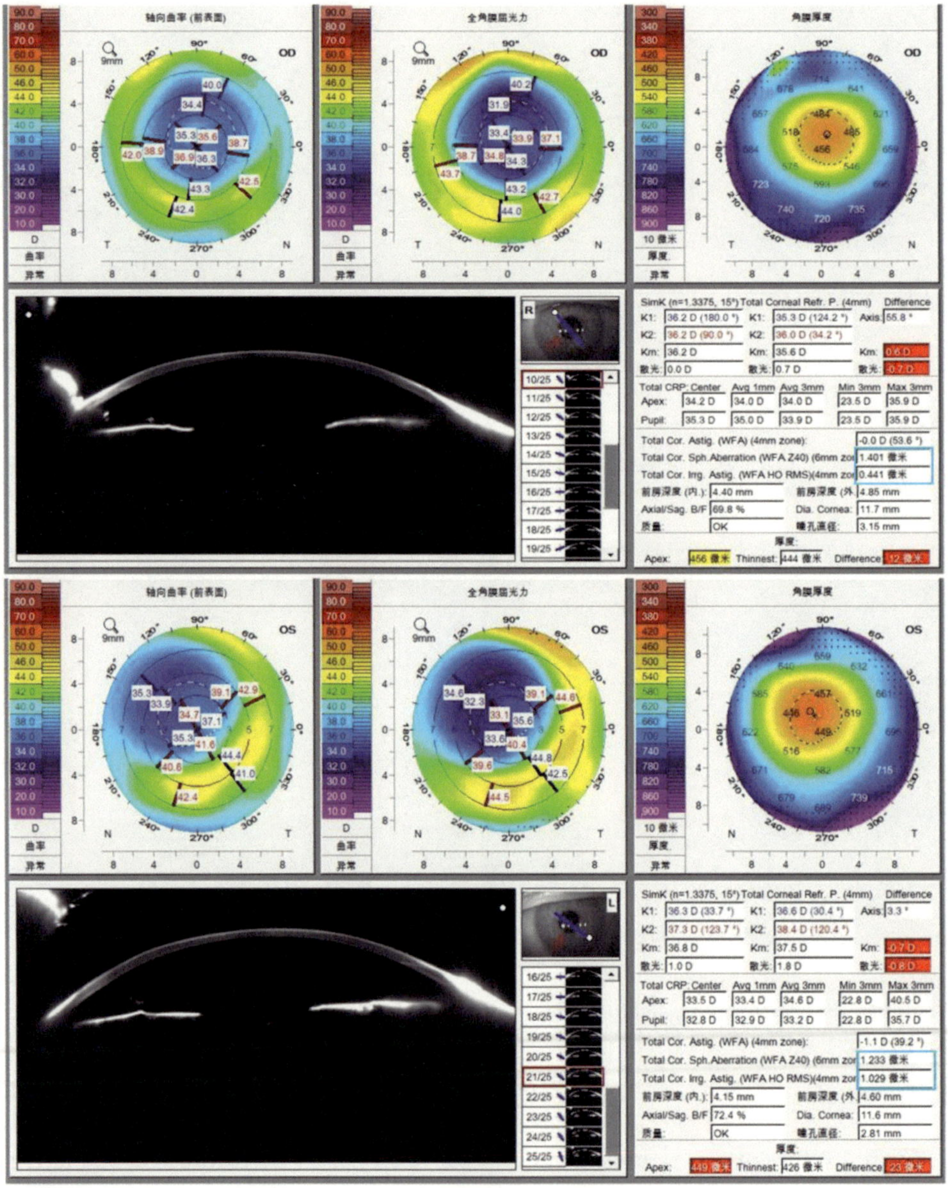

Figure 8.
A binocular Pentacam image taken on June 05, 2019, showing that corneal astigmatism, total corneal spherical aberration (SA), and total corneal irregular astigmatism are all reduced compared with those before surgery.

after a comprehensive preoperative evaluation, a symmetric clear corneal incision on a steep axis was used to correct corneal astigmatism. Pentacam examination after surgery showed that corneal astigmatism was corrected to a certain extent, and corneal irregular astigmatism and SA were reduced. This played a certain role in improving the visual quality of patients after surgery. The absence of evident symptoms of visual disturbance and discomfort after surgery in the patient may be related to the neurological adaptability of the brain for many years. Therefore, when the phacoemulsification cataract surgery removed the effects of cataract-induced refractive interstitial opacity and myopia and reduced astigmatism, irregularities, and SA, the patient had improved vision without the occurrence of any additional symptoms of visual disturbance and discomfort. For the calculation of IOL power, we used the formula for the calculation of IOL after myopic refractive surgery on the ASCRS website, took the average power as the final IOL power, and obtained a relatively accurate target refraction after the operation.

Through the analysis of this case, we can provide certain experience references for more patients who had undergone early myopia refractive surgery, particularly for some patients who desired to receive an implant of trifocal IOL but had decentered ablation, irregular corneal astigmatism, and large SA caused by early refractive surgery.

4. A case of early capsular shrinkage syndrome after cataract surgery for retinitis pigmentosa and high myopia eyes

On March 5, 2018, a patient with binocular retinitis pigmentosa and high myopia complicated with cataract was admitted to hospital. The visual acuity was hand motion in both eyes; intraocular pressure was 15 mmHg in the right eye and 20 mmHg in the left eye; there was alternating exotropia and nystagmus in both eyes. The lens cortex of the right eye had localized opacity, and the nucleus was opaque and dark brown; the left lens nucleus was opaque and brown-yellow, and there was obvious posterior subcapsular opacity (**Figure 9**).

The patient underwent small incision cataract extraction in the right eye and phacoemulsification cataract surgery in the left eye on March 8, 2018, and April 3, 2018, respectively. The author knew that both retinitis pigmentosa and high myopia are risk factors for capsular contraction syndrome (CCS), small incision cataract extraction in the right eye was performed gently and the continuous curvilinear capsulorhexis (CCC) diameter was larger than 6 mm; the patient's lens suspensory

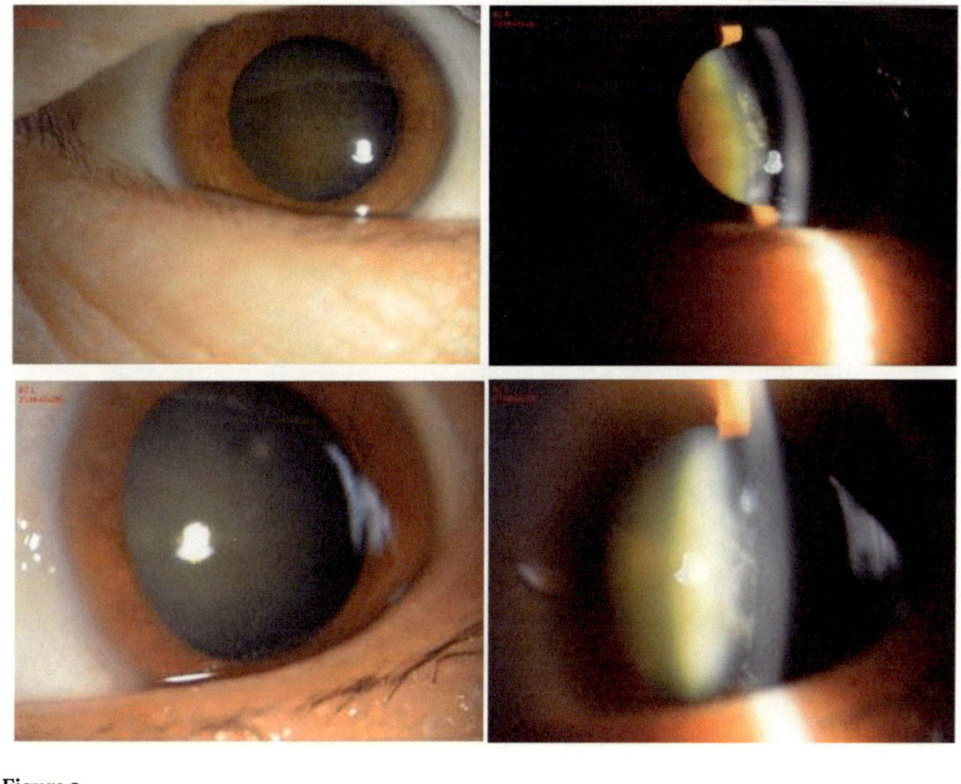

Figure 9.
The state of binocular lens opacity (the upper row is the right eye, and the lower row is the left eye).

ligament was found to loosen during capsulorhexis. When the residual cortex was aspirated, starfish-like cortical debris was found attached to the posterior capsule, which was polished using a viscoelastic needle. As the pupil could not be fully dilated, the IOL positioning hook assisted in the dilation of the pupil, the equatorial cortex was aspirated as far as possible, the posterior capsule was carefully polished, and finally, a one-piece hydrophilic acrylic IOL was implanted. Postoperative vision in the right eye was 0.2, intraocular pressure was 17 mmHg, the cornea was clear, pupils were round, light reflection was good, aqueous flare was ++, the IOL position was good, and retinitis pigmentosa and high myopic changes were observed in the fundus. The patient received prednisolone acetate eye drops 8 times a day and levofloxacin, pranoprofen, and 3% sodium hyaluronate eye drops four times a day. At the re-examination 1 week after the operation, the anterior chamber inflammation was significantly relieved, the IOL position was stable, the rest were similar to that at 1 day after surgery. The patient came to the hospital for scheduled cataract surgery for the left eye, 20 days after the operation. Re-examination showed right eye visual acuity as 0.25 and the intraocular pressure as 18 mmHg; the cornea was clear as revealed by the slit lamp examination, the aqueous flare was -, the pupils were round, and light reflection was good. Mydriatic examination showed that the anterior capsular opening was shrunk to less than 4 mm with obvious CCS (**Figure 10**).

CCS was quite obvious soon after cataract surgery, and timely detection and treatment were necessary to prevent serious complications. Therefore, after communicating with the patient, YAG laser anterior capsular opening lysis was performed for the right eye of the patient. First, the site of the anterior capsule with less tension was selected; then the anterior capsule was opened using laser, and the laser was used continuously at the contralateral site to loosen the shrunk anterior capsule, and the rest was performed in a manner similar to that followed to loosen the anterior capsule around the entire circumstance. It was forbidden to directly select the edge of the capsular opening for laser lysis, as asymmetrical dehiscence of the capsular membrane might occur due to excessive tension (**Figure 11**).

After YAG laser surgery, slit-lamp examination showed that the patient had more floating white crystalline cortical debris in the anterior chamber of the right eye. The intraocular pressure was 30 mmHg. He received prednisolone acetate eye drops four times a day; timolol eye drops two times/day; levofloxacin, pranoprofen,

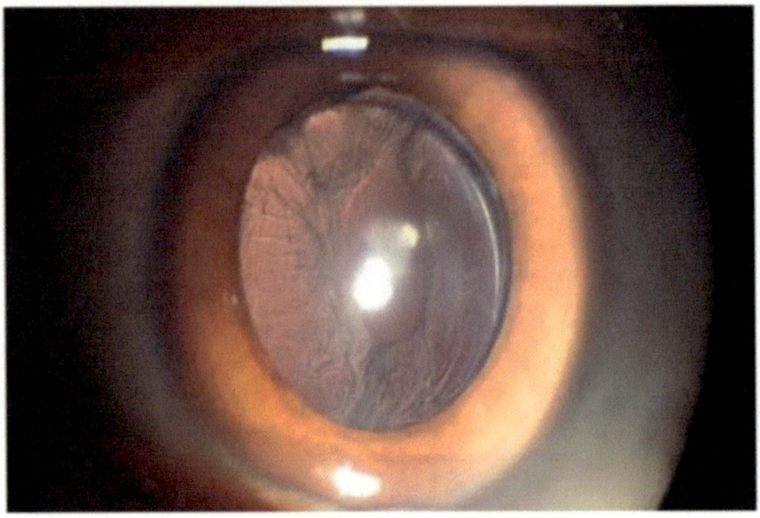

Figure 10.
Anterior capsular opening of the right eye is shrunk.

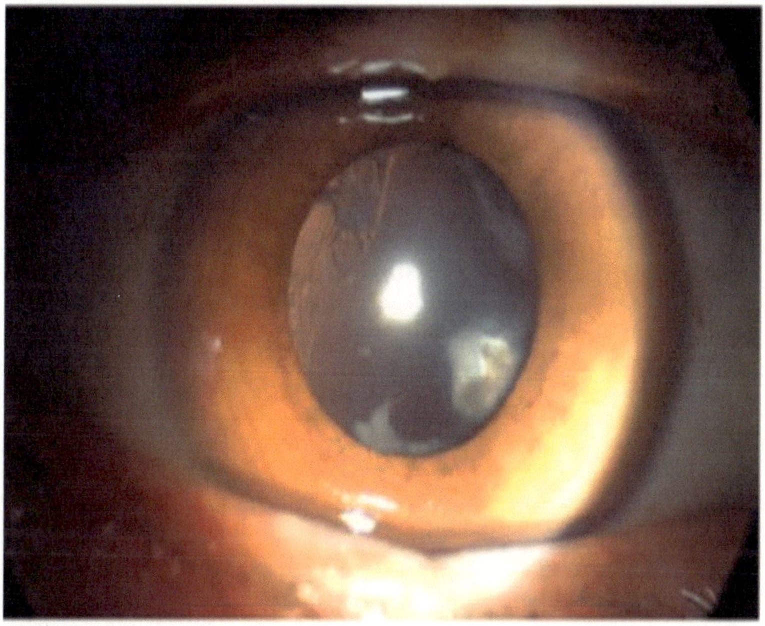

Figure 11.
The shrinkage of the anterior capsular opening is significantly reduced after laser lysis in the right eye.

and 3% sodium hyaluronate eye drops four times/day, and the patient was asked to visit for re-examination the next day. The re-examination showed that the visual acuity of the right eye was 0.25 and the intraocular pressure was 22 mmHg. The slit-lamp examination showed that the cortical debris floating in the anterior chamber of the right eye was significantly reduced, and the IOL position was stable. The patient was instructed to continue the medication and to visit for re-examination after 3 days. The re-examination showed the visual acuity of the right eye was 0.25, and the intraocular pressure was 17 mmHg. The slit-lamp examination showed only a small amount of floating cortical debris in the anterior chamber of the right eye, and the IOL position was stable; the patient was instructed to continue the previous medication. Because the degree of cataract in the left eye of the patient was lighter than that of the right eye and the nuclear hardness grade was lower than that of the right eye, phacoemulsification cataract aspiration in the left eye was scheduled on April 3, 2018. Owing to the experience in the right eye, special attention was paid to the prevention of CCS during the perioperative period of the left eye. First, preoperatively, non-steroidal anti-inflammatory drug pranoprofen eye drops were administered four times a day to reduce the intraoperative inflammation and maintain the dilated state of the pupil during the operation. Second, operations were performed as gently as possible during the surgery to reduce mechanical irritation to the iris to reduce the release of inflammatory mediators. During capsulorhexis, the suspensory ligament of the lens was loosened, and the diameter of the capsulorhexis opening was larger than 6 mm. Sufficient hydrodissection was performed to reduce the pulling effect of the intraoperative operation on the ligament, during the phacoemulsification process, the nucleus was split into smaller nuclei as far as possible before performing emulsification to reduce the release of ultrasound energy. When the emulsification was completed and the residual cortex was aspirated, the central part of the posterior capsule showed starfish-like attached cortical debris, which was tightly attached to the posterior capsule. It was mechanically polished using a viscoelastic needle, and the anterior subcapsular region was polished using a polisher around the whole circumference to reduce postoperative proliferation. A one-piece hydrophilic acrylate IOL of the same model was implanted. On the second day after surgery, re-examination showed that the left eye visual acuity was 0.3, and the intraocular pressure was 16 mmHg; the slit-lamp examination showed clear cornea, round pupils, good light reflection, aqueous flare was ++, and normal IOL position. The patient received prednisolone acetate eye drops eight times a day and levofloxacin, pranoprofen, and 3% sodium hyaluronate eye drops four times a day. The left eye was re-examined 20 days after surgery, the visual acuity was 0.3, the intraocular pressure was 18 mmHg, the cornea was clear, the aqueous flare was -, the pupil was round, and the light reflection was good. Mydriatic examination showed that the anterior capsular opening was shrunk, less than 4 mm, and CCS was evident. A YAG laser anterior capsule lysis was performed for the patient's left eye, and good postoperative results were achieved (**Figure 12**).

4.1 Discussion

This case study analyzed a case of a complicated cataract patient with binocular retinitis pigmentosa and high myopia who developed severe CCS short-term postoperatively, and both eyes were treated using YAG laser lysis.

Most of the capsular bag shrinkage caused by non-specific stimulation after cataract surgery occurs in the anterior lens capsule [20]. Residual lens epithelial cells (LEC) under the margin of the anterior capsule produce a variety of cytokines under the surgical stimulation and stimulation by different material IOLs. These factors may react against LEC and make it produce collagen and fibers through autocrine or paracrine, leading to shrinkage of the anterior capsular opening [21].

Several studies have shown that silicone gel IOLs have a higher incidence of CCS than other types of IOLs [22, 23]. The study of Tsinopoulos et al. [24] showed that hydrophilic acrylate IOL has a higher incidence of CCS than hydrophobic acrylate IOL. Although hydrophilic acrylic material has better uveal biocompatibility, lower adhesion of bacteria and silicone oil, and less incidence of glare, its weak adhesion to type IV collagen leads to an increased incidence of fibrosis, which is more likely to lead to the occurrence of CCS [25–27]. The hydrophobic acrylate IOL can inhibit the migration of LEC to the optical zone and loops, thereby reducing the occurrence of CCS [22, 28, 29]. In this case, both eyes of the patient used hydrophilic acrylic IOL, which may also be one of the risk factors for the rapid occurrence of CCS. Studies have shown that one-piece acrylate and three-piece acrylate IOL have similar incidences of CCS [30]. Another study showed that four-loop IOL is more effective in preventing postoperative IOL eccentricity and CCS [31].

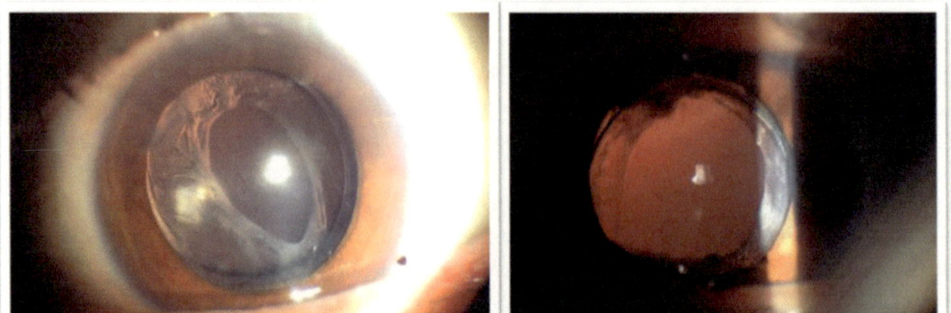

Figure 12.
Image of the capsular opening that was shrunk after the operation of the left eye. Image of the capsular opening that is in good condition after YAG laser anterior capsule lysis.

Studies have shown that the size of the diameter of capsulorhexis is closely related to CCS. CCC larger than 5.5 mm showed an increasing trend in the change of the size of the capsulorhexis after surgery; conversely, the capsulorhexis opening of CCC smaller than 5 mm showed a gradually shrinking trend after the surgery [32]. Anterior capsule opacity after cataract surgery occurs only in the part where the anterior capsule is in contact with the IOL. Therefore, the smaller the capsulorhexis diameter, the more obvious the anterior capsule opacity and organization will be, thereby aggravating the occurrence of capsular bag shrinkage. To prevent postoperative CCS, the diameter of the capsulorhexis, in this case, was greater than 6 mm; however, it did not have an obvious preventive effect. This may be related to other risk factors that are prone to CCS in the patient.

All diseases that easily affect the normal function of the suspensory ligament and lead to the fragility of the suspensory ligament are risk factors for the occurrence of CCS, including retinitis pigmentosa, high myopia, and advanced age [33]. The shrinkage area of the capsular bag of patients with retinitis pigmentosa was significantly larger than that of the normal control group, which was close to 25%. In total, 9.4% of the retinitis pigmentosa group underwent YAG laser anterior capsulotomy within 12 months after surgery. The anterior capsular opening area of these patients was all less than 10 mm^2 [34]. Diseases involving abnormal blood–aqueous barrier function, including exfoliation syndrome, uveitis, diabetes, and myotonic dystrophy, were all risk factors for CCS [35, 36]. The stimulation of cataract surgery is more likely to lead to the destruction of the barrier, thus causing the occurrence of CCS. Moreover, patients with diabetic retinopathy are more likely to develop CCS than those without fundus disease [35].

The treatment of CCS includes YAG laser anterior capsulotomy and surgical treatment. YAG laser is a safe and effective method for the treatment of early CCS, which can effectively enlarge the anterior capsule opening and restore visual function [37]. The study by Deokule et al. [37] showed that the success rate of YAG laser treatment of CCS was 78%, while the failure rate of preoperative IOL eccentric cases was high. Some researchers have reported [38, 39] that the early preventive application of YAG laser after cataract surgery for anterior capsulotomy at meridian 0°, 120°, and 240° can effectively prevent the occurrence of CCS in high-risk patients without adverse reactions. In more severe cases of CCS, YAG laser lysis cannot achieve effective treatment, and the proliferating fibrous membrane must be surgically seaparted under the anterior capsule and the adhesion of IOL edges and loops, to remove the fibrous membrane as far as possible by cutting or tearing it off. Radial cutting or direct continuous circular capsulorhexis was performed on the narrowed anterior capsular opening to remove the fibrous membrane, and there was no recurrence during postoperative follow-up [40]. Yeh et al. [41] proposed to use an anterior vitrectomy to cut the shrunk anterior capsular opening to remove the subcapsular fibrous membrane and residual lens epithelial cells, which can reduce the chance of radial tear of the suspensory ligament and secondary IOL eccentricity. The disadvantage of the surgical method is that it may cause further damage to the suspensory ligament and IOL eccentricity for patients with poor suspensory ligament function.

The prevention of CCS mainly includes the following aspects: (1) The application of preoperative non-steroidal anti-inflammatory drugs can effectively reduce the release of intraoperative inflammatory factors, thereby preventing the progression of anterior capsule shrinkage [42]. (2) Avoid excessive stimulation of the iris tissue and further aggravation of the destruction of the blood-aqueous barrier during whole operation. The diameter of the CCC should be 5.5–6.0 mm. The complete removal of the residual LEC under the anterior capsule helps to prevent the excessive proliferation of the anterior capsular opening, preventing CCS [43].

(3) Adequate anti-inflammatory treatment should be provided after the operation, which should be combined with glucocorticoid and non-steroidal anti-inflammatory eye drops, and the use time of non-steroidal anti-inflammatory drugs should be appropriately extended, which can effectively control the postoperative inflammatory response of operation and plays a role in preventing CCS. (4) In terms of IOL selection, hydrophobic acrylate materials are the first choice. (5) The use of intraoperative capsular tension ring. Studies have shown that the implantation of the capsular bag tension ring can effectively prevent IOL eccentricity, tilt, and significantly prevent capsular bag shrinkage [44, 45].

5. Conclusions

In conclusion, in actual clinical work, surgeons will encounter a variety of special conditions. Based on different conditions, the surgeon should comprehensively evaluate the surgical plan and the specific conditions before and after the operation, and deal with them in a targeted manner, to improve the post-operative visual quality of patients.

Acknowledgements

This work was supported by the National Natural Science Foundation of China under Grant No. 81971697, 81501544.

Conflict of interest

The authors declare no conflict of interest.

Notes/thanks/other declarations

None.

DOI: http://dx.doi.org/10.5772/intechopen.98260

Author details

Minghui Deng[1,2,3]*, Song Chen[1,2] and Xiaogang Wang[4]

1 Clinical College of Ophthalmology, Tianjin Medical University, Tianjin, China

2 Tianjin Eye Hospital, Tianjin Eye Institute, Tianjin Key Lab of Ophthalmology and Visual Science, Tianjin, China

3 Department of Cataract, Linfen Yaodu Eye Hospital, Linfen, Shanxi, P.R. China

4 Department of Cataract, Shanxi Eye Hospital, Taiyuan, Shanxi, P.R. China

*Address all correspondence to: 49332484@qq.com

References

[1] de Vries NE, Nuijts RM. Multifocal intraocular lenses in cataract surgery: literature review of benefits and side effects. J Cataract Refract Surg. 2013;39(2):268-78.

[2] Srinivasaraghavan, P., et al., *Extended focal length intraocular lens implantation in posttraumatic posterior capsular rupture.* Indian J Ophthalmol, 2018. **66**(5): p. 701-704.

[3] Lever J,Dahan E.Opposite clear corneal incision to correct pre-existing astigmatism in cataract surgery[J]. J Cataract Refract Surg,2000,26(6): 803-805.

[4] Chiam PJ.Effect of paired opposite clear corneal incision on with-the-rule versus against-the-rule astigmatism[J]. Cornea,2015,34(8):901-905. DOI:10.1097/ICO.0000000000000441.

[5] Nemeth G,Kolozsvari B,Berta A, et al. Paired opposite clear corneal incision:time-related changes of its effect and factors on which those changes depend[J]. Eur J Ophthalmol, 2014,24(5):676-681. DOI:10.5301/ejo.5000428

[6] Koch, D.D., et al., *Correcting astigmatism with toric intraocular lenses: effect of posterior corneal astigmatism.* J Cataract Refract Surg, 2013. **39**(12): p. 1803-9.

[7] Vasavada, A.R. and V.A. Vasavada, *Managing the posterior polar cataract: An update.* Indian J Ophthalmol, 2017. **65**(12): p. 1350-1358.

[8] Foster, G.J.L., et al., *Phacoemulsification of posterior polar cataracts.* J Cataract Refract Surg, 2019. **45**(2): p. 228-235.

[9] Vasavada, A.R., et al., *Surgical approaches to posterior polar cataract: a review.* Eye (Lond), 2012. **26**(6): p. 761-70.

[10] Duke-Elder S, editor. System of Ophthalmology 3, Pt. 2 Normal and Abnormal Development, Congenital Deformities. St. Louis, MO: CV Mosby; 1964. Posterior polar cataract; pp. 723-6.

[11] Iijima K, Kamiya K, Shimizu K, Igarashi A, Komatsu M. Demographics of patients having cataract surgery after laser in situ keratomileusis. J Cataract Refract Surg. 2015;41(2):334-8.

[12] Fernandez-Vega L, Madrid-Costa D, Alfonso JF, Montes-Mico R, Poo-Lopez A. Optical and visual performance of diffractive intraocular lens implantation after myopic laser in situ keratomileusis. J Cataract Refract Surg. 2009;35(5):825-32.

[13] Muftuoglu O, Dao L, Mootha VV, Verity SM, Bowman RW, Cavanagh HD, McCulley JP. Apodized diffractive intraocular lens implantation after laser in situ keratomileusis with or without subsequent excimer laser enhancement. J Cataract Refract Surg. 2010;36(11): 1815-21.

[14] Vrijman V, van der Linden JW, van der Meulen IJE, Mourits MP, Lapid-Gortzak R. Multifocal intraocular lens implantation after previous corneal refractive laser surgery for myopia. J Cataract Refract Surg. 2017;43(7):909-14.

[15] Chang JS, Ng JC, Chan VK, Law AK. Visual outcomes, quality of vision, and quality of life of diffractive multifocal intraocular lens implantation after myopic laser in situ keratomileusis: a prospective, observational case series. J Ophthalmol. 2017;2017:6459504.

[16] Mojzis P, Majerova K, Hrckova L, Pinero DP. Implantation of a diffractive trifocal intraocular lens: one-year follow-up. J Cataract Refract Surg. 2015;41(8):1623-30.

[17] Kohnen T, Titke C, Bohm M. Trifocal intraocular lens implantation to

treat visual demands in various distances following lens removal. Am J Ophthalmol. 2016;161:71-7.

[18] Wang W, Ni S, Li X, Chen X, Zhu Y, Xu W. Femtosecond laser-assisted cataract surgery with implantation of a diffractive trifocal intraocular lens after laser in situ keratomileusis: a case report. BMC Ophthalmol. 2018;18(1):160.

[19] Chow SSW, Chan TCY, Ng ALK, Kwok AKH. Outcomes of presbyopia-correcting intraocular lenses after laser in situ keratomileusis. Int Ophthalmol. 2019;39(5):1199-204.

[20] Andjelic S, Zupancic C, Perovsek D, et al. Human anterior lens capsule epithelial cells contraction. Acta Ophthalmol,2011,89:645-653.

[21] Nishi T, Nishi K. Intraocular lens encapsulation by shrinkage of the capsulorhexis opening. J Cataract Refract Surg,1993,19: 544-545.

[22] Richter-Mueksch S, Kahraman G, Amon M,et al. Uveal an capsular biocompatibility after implantation of sharp-edged hydrophilic acrylic, hydrophobic acrylic,and silicone intraocular lenses in eyes with pseudoexfoliation syndrome. J Cataract Refract Surg,2007,33:1414-1418.

[23] Sacu S, Menapace R, Buehl W, et al. Effect of intraocular lens design and material on fibrotic capsule opacification and capsulorrhexis contraction. J Cataract Refract Surg,2004,30: 1875-1882.

[24] Tsinopoulos IT, Tsaousis KT, Kymionis GD, et al. Comparison of anterior capsule contraction between hydrophobic and hydrophilic intraocular lens models.Graefes Arch Clin Exp Ophthalmol,2010, 248:1155-1158.

[25] Kramer S, Schröder AC, Bruckner K, et al. Subluxation of hydrophilic acrylate intraocular lenses due to massive capsular fibrosis. Ophthalmologe, 2010,107: 460-464.

[26] Abela-Formanek C, Amon M, Kahraman G, et al.Biocompatibility of hydrophilic acrylic,hydrophobic acrylic,and silicone intraocular lenses in eyes with uveitis having cataract surgery:Long-term follow-up. J Cataract Refract Surg,2011,37: 104-112.

[27] Malik A, Gupta N, Sood S. Capsular contraction syndrome following insertion of hydrophilic acrylic lens. Int Ophthalmol,2011,31:121-123.

[28] Zemaitiene R, Speckauskas M, Glebauskiene B, et al. Comparison of postoperative results after implantation of hydrophilic acrylic or hydrophobic acrylic intraocular lens: data of one-year prospective clinical study. Medicina (Kaunas),2008,44:936-943.

[29] Gauthier L, Lafuma A, Laurendeau C, et al. Neodymium: YAG laser rates after bilateral implantation of hydrophobic or hydrophili multifocal intraocular lenses: twenty-four month retrospective comparative study.J Cataract Refract Surg,2010,36:1195-1200.

[30] Hayashi K, Hayashi H. Intraocular lens factors that may affect anterior capsule contraction.Ophthalmology, 2005,112:286-292.

[31] Mingels A, Koch J, Lommatzsch A, et al. Comparison of two acrylic intraocular lenses with different haptic designs in patients with combined phacoemulsification and pars plana vitrectomy. Eye,2007,21:1379-1381.

[32] Joo CK, Shin JA, Kim JH. Capsular opening contracture after continuous curvilinear capsulorrhexis and intraocular lens implantation.J Cataract Refract Surg,1996,22:585-590.

[33] Kato S, Suzuki T, Hayashi Y, et al. Risk factors for contraction of the

anterior capsule opening.J Cataract Refract Surg,2002,28: 109-112.

[34] Sudhir RR, Rao SK. Capsulorhexis phimosis in retinitis pigmentosa despite capsular tension ring implantation.J Cataract Refract Surg, 2001,27:1691-1694.

[35] Kato S, Oshika T, Numaga J, et al.Anterior capsular contraction after cataract surgery in eyes of diabetic patients. Br J Ophthalmol, 2001,85:21-23.

[36] Garrott HM, Walland MJ, O'Day J. Recurrent posterior capsular opacification and capsulorhexis contracture after cataract surgery in myotonic dystrophy. Clin Experiment Ophthalmol,2004,32: 653-655.

[37] Deokule SP, Mukherjee SS, Chew CK. Neodymium: YAG laser anterior capsulotomy for capsular contraction syndrome. Ophthalmic Surg Lasers Imaging,2006, 37: 99-105.

[38] Hayashi K, Yoshida M, Nakao F, et al. Prevention of Anterior Capsule Contraction by anterior Capsule Relaxing Incisions with Neodymium:Yttrium-Aluminum-Garnet Laser. Am J Ophthalmol, 2008,146: 23-30.

[39] Hayashi K, Yoshida M, Hirata A, et al. Anterior capsule relaxing incisions with neodymium:YAG laser for patients at high-risk for anterior capsule contraction. J Cataract Refract Surg, 2011,37: 97-103.

[40] Panagopoulos A, Chalioulias K, Kirkby GR. A new approach in the surgical management of anterior capsular phimosis syndrome. Ophthalmic Res, 2009, 42:221-223.

[41] Yeh PC, Goins KM, Lai WW. Managing anterior capsule contraction by mechanical widening with vitrector-cut capsulotomy. J Cataract Refract Surg, 2002,28:217-220.

[42] Mukai K, Matsushima H, Gotoh N, et al. Efficacy of ophthalmic nonsteroidal antiinflammatory drugs in suppressing anterior capsule contraction and secondary posterior capsule opacification. J Cataract Refract Surg,2009,35:1614-1618.

[43] Hanson RJ, Rubinstein A, Sarangapani S, et al. Effect of lens epithelial cell aspiration on postoperative capsulorhexis contraction with the use of the AcrySof intraocular lens: randomized clinical trial. J Cataract Refract Surg,2006,32:1621-1626.

[44] Kurtz S, Krummenauer F, Dumbach C, et al. Effect of a closed foldable equator ring on capsular bag shrinkage in cataract surgery. J Cataract Refract Surg,2006,32:1615-1620.

[45] Takimoto M, Hayashi K, Hayashi H. Effect of a capsular tension ring on prevention of intraocular lens decentration and tilt and on anterior capsule contraction after cataract surgery. Jpn J Ophthalmol,2008,52: 363-367.

Chapter 5

Visual Impairment Caused by Monovision Surgical Design

Humberto Dória Silva, Rostan Silvestre da Silva,
Eduardo Dória Silva, Maria Tamires Dória Silva,
Cristiana Pereira Dória and Cristiane Pereira Dória

Abstract

Neurophysiological anatomy of natural binocular vision shows the need to focus with both eyes to jointly produce the two corneas accommodation, correcting, in a compensatory way, the divergences inherent in the two different images, of the same visual field projected in the two distinct spaces, the two retinas. Corneal accommodation is part of the forced convection mechanism for the transfer of mobile mass in the cornea, trabecular meshwork and retina, to inhibit the accumulation of dehydrated intraocular metabolic residue, which can cause refractive errors in the cornea, obstruction of the trabecular meshwork and reduction of the amplitude of the signals produced by the phototransducers and sent to the brain. The IOL monovision surgical implantation technique differs from the physiology of natural binocular vision, which can cause after surgery disorders, described in this chapter, in that it imposes a different adaptation from the neurophysiological anatomy of human vision in addition to favoring the continuous progression of residue accumulation dehydrated intraocular metabolic and stimulate ocular.

Keywords: IOL monovision, binocular vision, corneal accommodation, corneal topography, forced convection, matabolic residue, stereoscopy

1. Introduction

This work is part of the research group "Mass transfer in flexible porous medium" certified by the Federal University of Pernambuco - UFPE at the National Council for Scientific and Technological Development – CNPq, of the Ministério da Ciência, Tecnologia e Inovações (Ministry of Science, Technology and Innovation), of the Federal Government of Brazil. Physically, a flexible porous medium can be a cleaning sponge but it can serve as a model to demonstrate the mass transfer movement by forced convection in the cornea, lens, trabecular meshwork and retina, as well as muscles.

In the research it was found that in the experiments carried out by the German astronomer and Jesuit Christoph Scheinerque, in 1619, *apud* [1], with holes in a card, when observing the same object through different holes, different distances are perceived, corresponding to the intraocular lenses formed by dehydrated metabolic residue droplets [2]. That is, the card selects the image to be viewed in an overlay of images, which may be the astigmatism cause, in addition to myopia or hyperopia [3].

The research group leader exercises his own eyes to solve his eye refraction problems and discusses with the researchers group the understanding of the intraocular process of dehydration and rehydration of metabolic residue.

In this chapter we will show that the implantation technique known as IOL monovision, should be performed only if the patient accepts the act, after being informed, in writing, of the possible negative consequences that may occur to his health following cataract surgery. The difficulties in living with the symptoms acquired by a patient submitted to this surgical technique are presented, as well as the preoperative exams. Before surgery the patient was authorized by the doctor to renew his driver's license to drive motor vehicles without the use of corrective lenses.

2. Binocular oculomotricity

Rectus muscles: Maintain the central fixation point, the intersection of the visual axes, projected in the respective central ocular fovea [2].

Superior oblique muscle: [2] Controls the cylindrical corneal dioptric power that is part of the moving mass transfer mechanism of the cornea and retina by forced convection and moves the trabecular meshwork to prevent obstructing the passage of aqueous humor [4]. The cerebral hemisphere adjusts the projected image on the contralateral eye nasal retina to the projected image on the ipsilateral eye temporal retina by contralateral eye superior oblique muscle contraction or relaxation, with the help of the other muscles to prevent torsional movement of the contralateral eye, so if the technician positions the corneal topography equipment without the contralateral eye occlusion then when turning off the light used for positioning the equipment the projected image on the contralateral eye temporal retina ceases to exist and can cause superior oblique muscle relaxation and repositioning of the eye under examination.

Inferior oblique muscle: Has antagonistic action to the torsional force of the superior oblique muscle to prevent cyclotorsional movement of the eye [2].

Ciliary muscle: controls the lens accommodation to select the depth of focus and moves its moving mass [2, 4].

Iris: Reduce the light diffusion in the projected image in the retina and prevents aqueous humor return when the pressure in the anterior chamber is greater than in the posterior one during the natural process of corneal cylindrical diopter power variation due to the images fusion [3–5].

Binocular visual field: It is the intersection of the visual fields of the two eyes. The person can focus on the tip of a pencil placed over the nasal root, this being the limit of near vision.

Retina: Its main function is to discretize the analog image projected on its photoreceptors, transduce it into neural signals and send them to the respective hemispheres.

3. Neurophysiological anatomy of natural binocular vision

3.1 Physioanatomy in the writing movement

To facilitate the explanation of the importance of the movement of the superior oblique muscle, the writing of a person covering a calligraphic text was chosen [2]. The superior oblique muscle, when accommodating the cornea, moves the forced intraocular convection mechanism, which keeps the mobile mass in agitation to prevent the accumulation of dehydrated metabolic residue. Due to personal habits, the forced convection mechanism is impaired and the oculomotor system starts to accumulate dehydrated metabolic residue in droplet form [2], so the older the person, the greater the amount of droplets stored and the less visual acuity. This is the inducing reason why many believe in the link between age and visual degradation.

Figure 1a was created to explain the connection of the observed visual field and its relationship with the interpretation of the image. **Figure 1a** corresponds to one of the forms used by a right-handed person, with natural vision, when covering a calligraphic text. The visual axes of both eyes converge at the tip of the pencil, so the dashed vertical line which passes at the tip of the pencil divides the writer's visual field into the right and left visual fields. The right and left visual fields are projected inverted on the retinas of both eyes, **Figure 1b**, however, on the temporal retinas of their respective contralateral eye and on the nasal retinas of their respective ipsilateral eye. Optical discs are part of their respective nasal retina, that is, the projections on the two temporal retinas are more accurate than their respective projections on the nasal retinas.

The image projected onto the temporal retina, **Figure 1b**, is transduced to its respective ipsilateral cerebral hemisphere, **Figure 1c2**, and the image projected onto the nasal retina, **Figure 1b**, is transduced to its respective contralateral cerebral hemisphere, **Figure 1c2**.

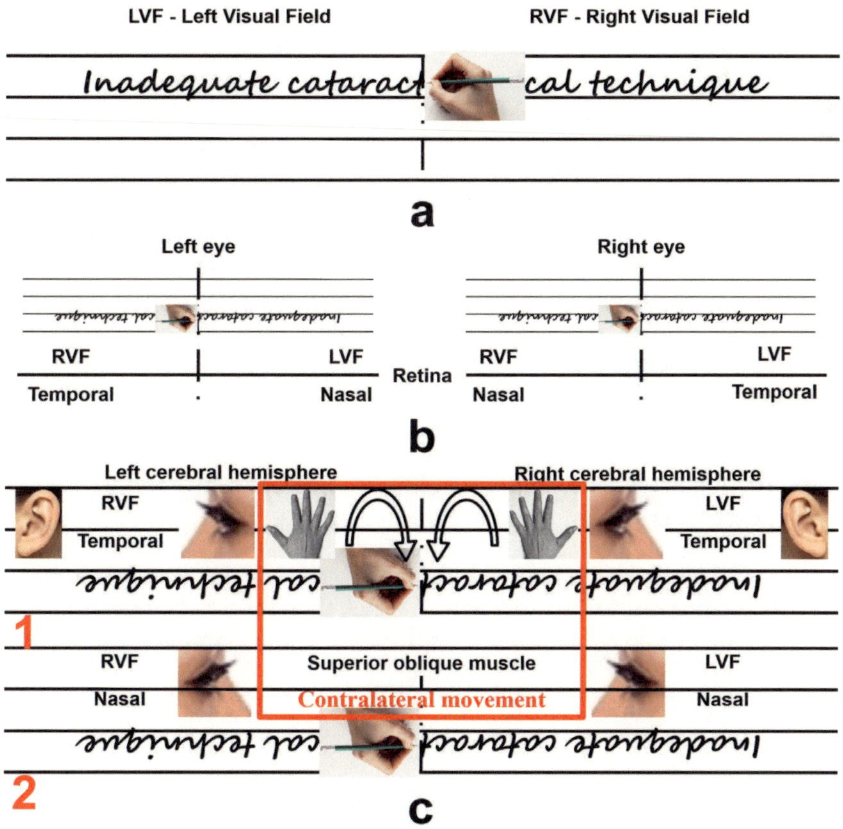

Figure 1.
Diagram showing the projection of the image on the retina and its transduction to the brain. (a) Visual fields, (b) projection into the human eye, (c) image sent to the brain, 1 - ipsilateral transduction, 2 - contralateral transduction.

Then, each cerebral hemisphere receives ipsilateral hearing and the projected image on the temporal retina of the ipsilateral eye, and, if it exists, includes the image of the contralateral hand, **Figure 1c1**, in addition to receiving the image projected on the nasal retina of the contralateral eye, and, if it exists, it includes the image of the ipslateral hand, **Figure 1c2**.

Each cerebral hemisphere controls, the contralateral superior oblique muscle, **Figure 1c2** and all other ipsilateral eye muscles (the rectus, inferior oblique, ciliary, iris, superior eyelid lift), control the movements of the contralateral hand and the rotating movement of the head in the contralateral direction **Figure 1c1**.

3.2 Eye exercises

The same interpretation of the oculomotor action of writing covering a calligraphic text, exposed through the diagram shown in **Figure 1**, is used in the analysis of the focus of a person's gaze, at the lateral limit of his binocular vision, the tip of the finger of his hand, very near to the nasal root, **Figure 2**, as children do in their initial oculomotor development. In **Figure 2a**, the right eye is diagrammed, positioning its visual axis tangent to the nasal root and intercepting the visual axis of the contralateral eye at a focus point common to both eyes, on the middle finger, of the contralateral hand, and on the **Figure 2b**, the left eye is diagrammed, positioning its visual axis tangent to the nasal root and intercepting the visual axis of the contralateral eye at a focus point common to both eyes, on the middle finger, of the contralateral hand. So:

- Ocular dominance, whether natural or pathological, fuses the images and alternates the dominant eye. As strabismus refers to eye misalignment [6], there can be no fusion of images or alternation in eye dominance, but surgical correction of strabismus is performed to restore or reconstruct normal eye alignment, to obtain normal visual acuity in each eye and be able to improve image fusion [6], then the patient can recover the alternating ocular dominance.

- The natural ocular dominance of the right eye, **Figure 2a**, and the left eye, **Figure 2b**, have their motor control image projected on the contralateral eye nasal retina, because in their ipsilateral temporal retina no image is projected. Thus, the contralateral cerebral hemisphere adjusts the greatest contraction of its superior oblique muscle, just as it adjusts the greatest contraction of the non-dominant eye natural lens, with its superior oblique muscle having the least contraction.

- By protecting newborns' nails with gloves to prevent injury these children miss the opportunity to adjust eye control.

- In the positions shown in **Figure 2**, the contraction of the twelve oculomotor muscles is constant, for any distance of focus, therefore, it is an extremely important position to adjust the refractive power of the non-dominant eye natural lens.

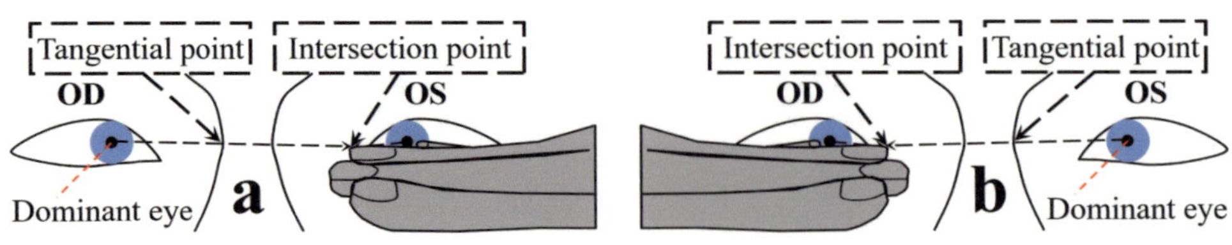

Figure 2.
Diagram showing the lateral limits of the binocular visual field. (a) left binocular limit, (b) right binocular limit.

4. Cataract surgery with monovision IOL

4.1 Etiopathogenesis of monovision

As [7] in monovision one eye (usually the dominant eye) is corrected for distance and the other eye is corrected for reading and according to [8] a lens set to far distances is implanted in your dominant eye, while a lens set to near distances is implanted in your non-dominant eye. It works because your brain automatically adjusts your visual system to achieve clear vision when you are focusing on near and distant objects [8].

This surgical technique uses pathological ocular dominance to maintain it and does not encourage its correction. In [2] it was demonstrated that in natural binocular vision, ocular dominance is alternated between the two eyes. But in [9] it says "If a strong degree of dominance is not apparent in a dominant eye test, it's more likely a person has mixed ocular dominance (*also called alternating ocular dominance*), where one eye is dominant for certain functions or tasks, and the other eye is dominant at different times", in addition to citing two criteria to determine ocular dominance, but under the hypothesis of alternating ocular dominance, that is, it identifies the natural ocular dominance acting alternately in both eyes.

In the work development, in the research group, it was found that in a simple frontal photo, a selfie, it is possible to perceive the result of pathological ocular dominance, but it is necessary to be sure that the photo is really frontal [10], see photo of **Figure 3**, because vicious ocular dominance can cause slight ocular deviation. Another way is to focus on the pencil tip that moves slowly to the nose root. The eye that keeps focusing on the pencil tip is the the dominant eye and the contralateral eye moves away quickly in its temporal direction, losing the focus point is the non-dominant eye, because who has natural binocular vision keeps both eyes focused on the pencil tip until it reaches the root of the nose effortlessly. The pathological ocular dominance is known as ocular dominance and in this chapter it is addressed only in its connections in planning and sequelae related to monovision surgery.

If a person, with one eye, sees the nearby objects well and with the contralateral eye sees the distant objects well, this situation was built through the convenience and personal habits, that is why, in this chapter, it is called ocular dominance, which is constructed involving eye shape and movement, in addition to the construction of neural communication, therefore, its surgical reproduction is impossible without the possibility of binocular vision. In this chapter, ocular dominance after monovision surgery is called dichotomous ocular dominance. Considering scientific knowledge, two surgical options are presented only for comparison with monovision surgery:

- **Bilateral monofocal intraocular lenses**: In this chapter it is considered that there are two monofocal lenses so that the eyes can focus on distant objects, although corrective lenses are required for reading. In this case, the distant focus is a known operational state of equilibrium, analogous to the state existing before surgery, and for reading, it is a state of temporary equilibrium, because of the use of corrective lenses, but both eyes focus simultaneously on same distance in both equilibrium states as well as images fusion.

- **Bilateral bifocal intraocular lenses**: In this chapter, it is considered that there are two lenses with two distinct optical powers so that the eyes can focus on far and near distant objects without the use of corrective lenses. In this case, the far focus and the near one are two well-known operational states of equilibrium, analogous to their corresponding states existing before the operation, because the two eyes simultaneously focus on common distances at different times.

Figure 3.
The four rectangles are equal to two. Dominant left eye, greater nasal distance [10].

It is very important to point out that the eye projections are conical consequently the visual field perimeter for near focusing is much smaller than the visual field perimeter for distant focusing, therefore the cylindrical diopter due to the images fusion is greater for near focusing, as was verified in [11]. It should be noted that the opposite reactions in 5 cases mentioned can be explained by the probable differences in the distribution of accumulated metabolic residue as presented in [12]. It is important to consider this diopter variation when calculating the lens power for focusing at near distances. This dioptric variation is important for the forced convection mechanism in the cornea and retina, in addition to moving the trabecular meshwork, thus it is an important option to be chosen.

After monovision cataract surgery there is no balance state because it is impossible to fuse images at near or distant focusing distances, causing a complete dichotomy difficult to overcome.

4.2 Case report

A 69 years old female patient in Recife, Brazil, who underwent, in June 2019, cataract surgery in the left eye with implantation of the LW 625A lens power + 24.00 [13], with near focus. **Table 1** shows the corrective lenses used by the patient who, despite having a lens prescribed before the surgery, but that patient did not need corrective lenses to renew the national driver's license three months before the surgery and the **Figure 4** shows the chronology of the examinations performed. In November 2020 the situation came to a stable discomfort. There is no solution, through the patient's health plan, because all the professionals who examine her report that the surgeon's work was very good, there was good healing and the lens very well positioned, it seems to be describing a work of art, but at the being asked about headaches, the health plan ophthalmologists, inform that there is nothing to do with the surgery and that the patient must have another problem and should seek another specialist, such as a neurologist, to know the source of the pain, because the surgery is perfect.

Preoperative: The patient can choose between a national or imported prosthesis, for an additional fee, but did not inform the origin of the lens. The patient filled out a form informing social life and answering about the lifestyle after surgery, without any explanation of the result of the choice:

1. Do not wear glasses near.
2. Do not wear glasses neither far nor near (patient's choice).
3. It does not matter whether or not to wear glasses.
4. Do not wear glasses away.

Based on the patient's response, the surgeon defines the solution without informing the patient of the result found.

It is devoid of logic for someone to seek the help of a professional to obtain a lower quality of life. On the other hand, when there are several alternatives for cataract surgery with an IOL implant, the choice of treatment must be given to the patient, given that it is the patient who will live with the consequences of the surgery.

Note	Rx.	Spherical		Cylindrical		Axis	
		O.D.	O.S.	O.D.	O.S.	O.D.	O.S.
Before surgery	D.V.	+0.75	+1.50	−0.75	−0.25	123°	170°
	N.V.	+3.00		add		—	
After surgery	D.V.	0.00	−2.25	−0.25	−1.50	41°	118°
	N.V.	+3.00		add		—	
Currently	D.V.	−0.75	−3.00	—		—	
	N.V.	+3.00		add		—	

Table 1.
Lenses prescribed by doctors.

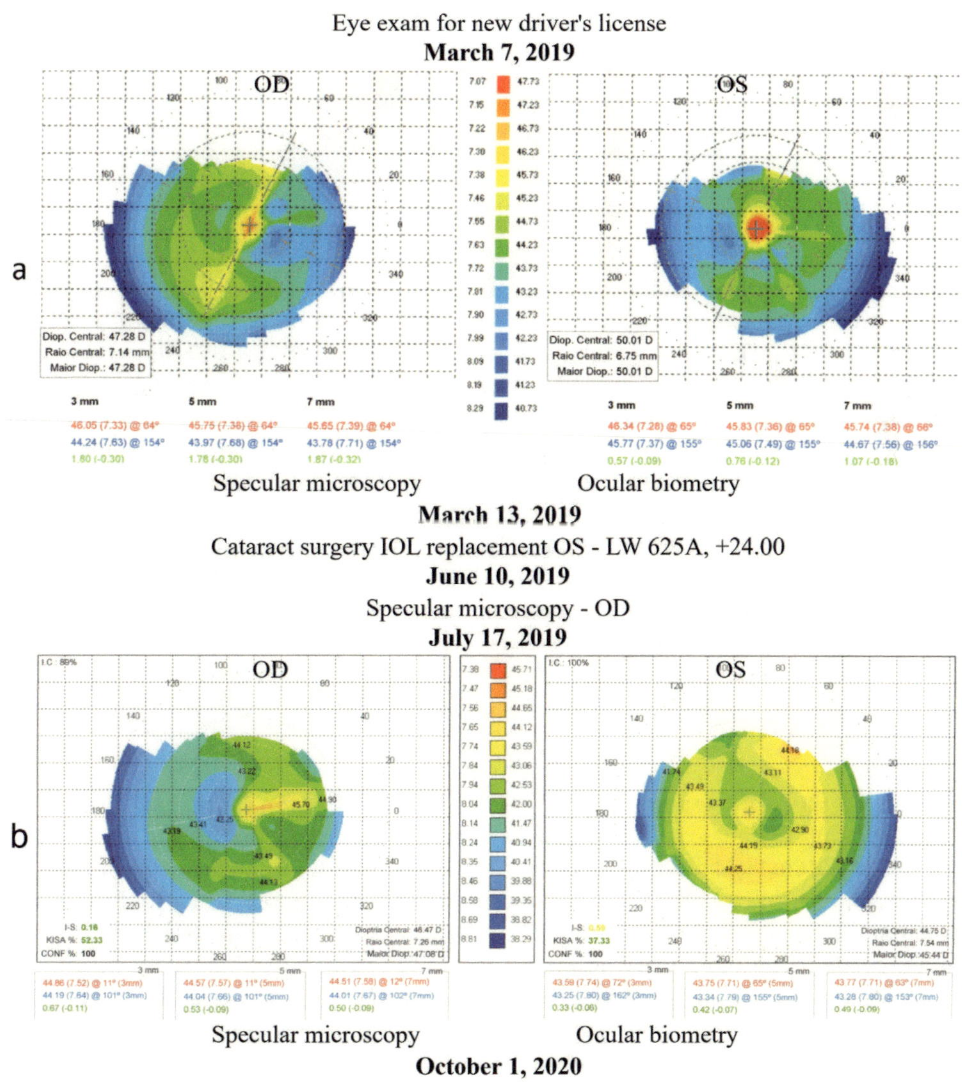

Figure 4.
History of exams performed by the patient. (a) before surgery, (b) after surgery.

Figure 4 shows the chronology of the surgery and exams, in addition to simulated keratometry of the corneas before, **Figure 4a**, and after, **Figure 4b**, surgery. The anterior corneal surface of the left eye, after surgery, is more regular

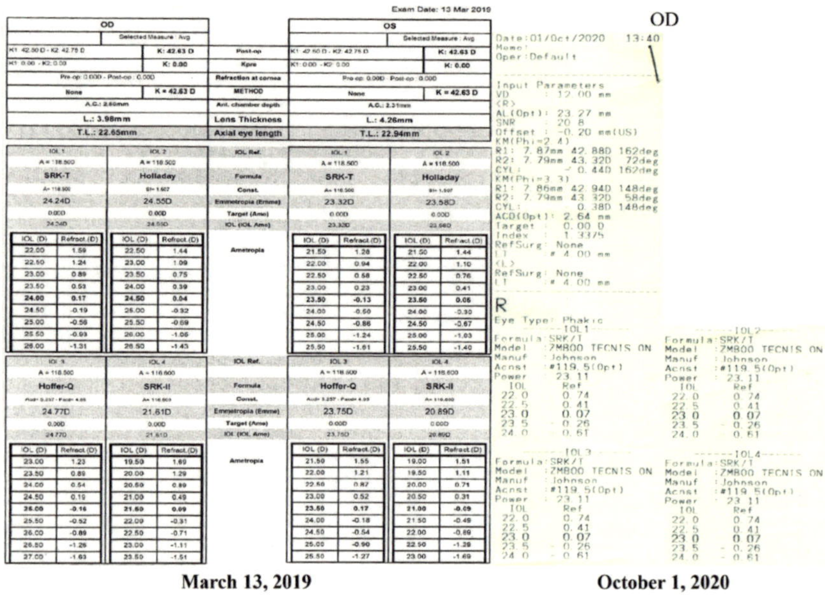

Figure 5.
Biometry before and after surgery.

than before the surgery and also in relation to the contralateral eye. The anterior surface of the cornea became more regular, As already explained in several studies [12, 14–16], the intraocular metabolic residue is dehydrated and stored, making a volume with high viscosity. To eliminate this viscous volume, it is necessary, first, to rehydrate it in order to reduce the viscosity and homogenize its concentration in the mobile mass, however, the only intraocular natural rehydration process available is the agitation performed through corneal flexion [14] using images fusion. In the 69-year-old patient case, the surgery made impossible for her to fuse the images, so there is no way to eliminate the metabolic residues from the cornea significantly. **Figure 5** shows the ocular biometry before and after surgery and **Figure 6** shows the specular microscopy before and after surgery, to better understand the patient's before and after operative conditions.

5. Conclusion

This chapter aims to show that there is no scientific reason for the use of the called monovision surgical technique, as well as to show that there are at least two scientific surgical alternatives. Two ways of ocular dominance are described, natural and pathological. Natural ocular dominance occurs according to the ocular system neurophysiological anatomy. Pathological ocular dominance is described in two forms, acquired and dichotomous. Acquired ocular dominance is known as ocular dominance and dichotomous ocular dominance, as referred to in this chapter, is characterized by surgical imposition. The three ocular dominances are described by their main functional characteristics and their consequences.

1. **Etiology of natural ocular dominance** - This ocular dominance is alternated between the eyes, so the dominate eye is the contralateral to the direction of the eye movement in relation to the head, its fixation, to reach an objective or to remain focused on a known objective, right after that, the dominant eye will be its contralateral one. This alternation of domination stimulates mainly the

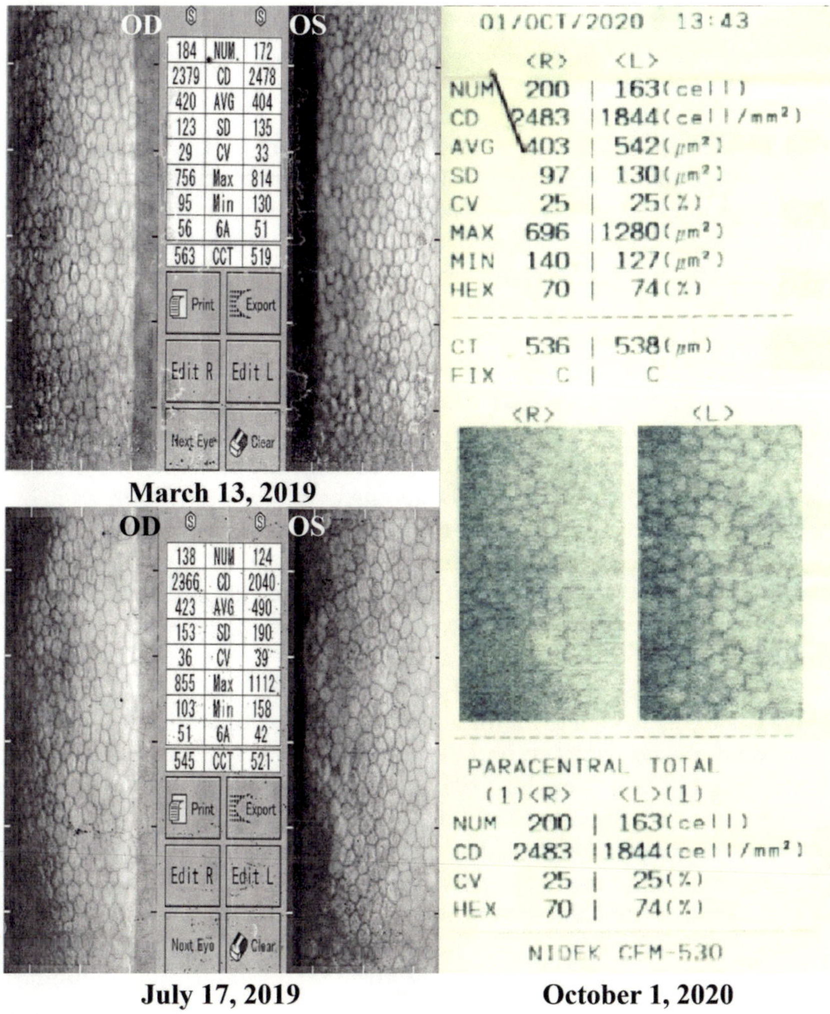

Figure 6.
Specular microscopy before and after surgery.

physiological process characteristic of the action of the two superior oblique muscles. The superior oblique muscle action changes the corneal cylindrical dioptric power and sustains the sclera in opposition to the consequent variation in intraocular pressure. Then, the cornea shape change is part of the mass movement forced convection mechanism in the cornea and retina, in addition to moving the trabecular meshwork, to avoid obstructing the passage of aqueous humor. Forced convection in the cornea and retina prevents the accumulation of metabolic residue that causes refractive error in the cornea and stiffens the retina. The ocular domain alternation is a fast process and makes small changes in the natural lens dioptric power that is part of its own forced convection mechanism to prevents the metabolic residues accumulation that cause refractive error and consequent opacity.

2. **Etiopathogenesis of ocular dominance** - This ocular dominance is the result of habits that are harmful to the intraocular forced convection mechanism. Then, the refractive error caused by the dehydrated metabolic residues accumulated in the cornea, retina and lens resist the natural movement of the eyes and create vicious pathological movements, such as the saccadic movement

[17] and the cyclotorsion movement mentioned in [18]. Dominance may not be full, as mentioned in [9], dominance depends on the evaluation criteria and usually for a specific activity.

3. **Etiopathogenesis of dichotomous ocular dominance** - This ocular dominance is the surgical result of imposing a lens set to far distances is implanted in your dominant eye, while a lens set to near distances is implanted in your non-dominant eye [8]. Thus, the patient is obliged to use corrective lenses in order to take advantage of his precarious intraocular force convection mechanism, before operative, however, upon waking up or when opening the eye during sleep, it causes an important impact, as it is not common to sleep with glasses, that is, the patient's brain spent 69 years adopting the direction of eye movement in relation to the head as a criterion for alternating ocular dominance and, due to the imposition of monovision surgery, in a "magic step", the focusing distance became the criterion for alternating ocular dominance without causing any disturbance for the patient. It is an alternative that should only be adopted with the permission given by the patient, after all, it is the patient who will be responsible for the administration of the after operative problems. In the case of the patient in focus, ocular dominance was imposed by the professional without the patient's knowledge, causing visual losses in precision, sharpness, agility, expansion, among others.

    - **Precision**: In [8] it is written that the patient may still need a pair of glasses to read small print for a few hours or to thread the needle. In the binocular view, each cerebral hemisphere receives the image projected on the temporal retina of the ipsilateral eye and simultaneously receives the image projected on the nasal retina of the contralateral eye, that is, for the more precise region of the retina, both eyes transmit neural signals twice as much to the brain, then, binocular vision is more than twice as accurate as monocular vision, with occlusion of one eye, since, in addition to having twice as many points, they are adjusted together, by the action of the superior oblique muscles, **Figure 1c**. This description combines with human perception, two eyes see better than one eye. The lack of precision is analogous to the sportsman using the sight out of alignment.
      The use of bilateral monofocal lenses maintains visual accuracy before surgery however one may need glasses for some activities.

    - **Sharpness**: In [8] it is written that the patient may still need a pair of glasses for nighttime driving. Analyzing **Figure 1c**, the monovision, without occlusion of the contralateral eye, is less clear, because a cerebral hemisphere receives the focused image projected on the temporal retina of the ipsilateral eye adding, as noise, without focusing, the image projected on the nasal retina of the contralateral eye and the contralateral cerebral hemisphere, receives, in focus, the image projected on the nasal retina of the contralateral eye to this cerebral hemisphere, without the region projected on its optic disc, adding, as noise, without focusing, the image projected on the temporal retina of the ipsilateral eye, that is, the patient's brain starts to receive the image focused by one eye with the addition of the defocused image of the contralateral eye. This is a form of stimulus for night blindness. The lack of sharpness is analogous to the sportsman who uses the target in smoke.
      The use of bilateral monofocal lenses can superimpose images with the same dimensions increasing the neural energy transmitted to the brain however one may need glasses for some activities.

- **Agility**: It is misleading to admit that the depth is given by binocular vision. If the depth depended on the simultaneous vision of the two eyes, the chicken would not be able to choose the grain of corn it eats. Animals that see their goal simultaneously with both eyes have greater agility of depth distance. The perception of distance depends on movement so astronomers are able to observe and analyze the universe with a telescope because there are movements. Those who have a natural binocular vision cannot visualize movements in static images nor can they view the stereoscopic image from photographs taken at two different points, they see two planes of images. When fixing an observation point, the alternation speed of the domain between the eyes produces dioptric powers changes in the crystallines for the rapid perception of depth but this visualization of depth is only possible up to a certain distance, from which, the brain makes use of the corneas diopter variation and for greater distances the person makes use of the head movement. After the monocular surgery there is no adjustment movement between the eyes and this may have been one of the causes of the 69 year patient's suffering. The substitution of the corneal movements for the movement of the head for depth perception the patient loses in agility because the corneas are more agile that the head, so the patient can be deprived of practicing activities that depend on agility and in transit may even cause an accident [19]. With dichotomous ocular dominance the patient may have difficulty to drive a motor vehicle, ride a bicycle and practice many sports such as tennis, ping pong, since in addition to the loss of agility, the brain receives the blurred image [20] of the contralateral eye. The lack of agility is analogous to that of sportsman with heavier equipment. An easy way to perceive the severity of the distance change problem is to use the basic principle observed by Scheinerque, in 1619, apud [1] through the using of pinhole glass [21] playing ping pong. One must be very careful when testing. The use of bilateral monofocal lenses maintains the mechanism of forced convection in the cornea, in the retina and the movement of the trabecular meshwork, fundamental for eye health, in addition to contributing to the perception of depth and has a much better result than that obtained with monovision surgery, however it may be necessary to wear glasses for some activities.

- **Dimension**: The monocular visual field has less visual space than the visual field with both eyes. No explanation is necessary but the monocular visual field blinds part of the contralateral eye's temporal visual field. The reduction of visual space is analogous to the sportsman located on the side of the wall.
  The use of bilateral monofocal lenses maintains the same dimensions of the visual field before surgery, however, one may need glasses for some activities.

To enable alternating ocular dominance if the surgery is bilateral bifocal the patient does not need corrective lenses and if the surgery is bilateral monofocal the patient must use near corrective lenses and if the surgery is monovision the patient must use two distinct optical powers of lenses.

The vision has many secrets as nobody knows how the other sees besides nobody can compare alternatives to intraocular lenses therefore if the patient is in a very adverse situation in his vision many of the basic movements he has already lost then any improvement is profit. This was not the 69 years old patient's situation before surgery. Monovision surgery only serves to prove the human being's adaptive power to stay alive.

After monofocal surgery, the patient cannot, without the use of corrective lenses, drive her vehicle or walk on the street safely [19, 20], in addition to losing the image fusion, blurred image [20] and, consequently, exposing herself to macular degeneration [15, 16], the increase in intraocular pressure (glaucoma) [2, 5, 10, 12] and, with corrective lenses, the 69-year-old patient suffers discomfort for read and headaches, today she prefers to abstain of read because of the great visual discomforts.

Monovision surgery and bilateral monofocus surgery do not interfere in the surgeon's fees or in the surgical costs of the clinic or health plan, in addition to not interfering in the values negotiated by the implanted lenses, so monovision surgery does not bring any financial advantage and can bring unrecoverable damage to the patient, why, in secret for the patient, use monovision surgery without any scientific basis?

Acknowledgements

To God for having helped the first author, in troubles during many years of suffering that led him to become an analytical observer of events in his own body, because of his mother, under the doctor's permission, 15 days before the birth of the first author, traveled by plane. In addition, by helping us to live, long ago, with the hardships as a result of internal political and economic decisions. For Marcos, first and third authors' brother, who saw in 1999 in a self-help book the importance of oculomotor muscle relaxation for eyesight treatment. To colleagues of the first author ANDES-SN Sindicato Nacional members and its Seção Sindical ADUFEPE members who during the intervals of same these organizations' meetings, provided important scientific information for the study. To those who were interviewed, friends, colleagues and family members who directly or indirectly have contributed to this work. To the engineer Florisnaldo Hermínio da Fonseca for the financial help in publishing this chapter. The authors agree with the individual mentions.

Author details

Humberto Dória Silva[1*], Rostan Silvestre da Silva[2], Eduardo Dória Silva[1], Maria Tamires Dória Silva[3], Cristiana Pereira Dória[4] and Cristiane Pereira Dória[5]

1 Federal University of Pernambuco - UFPE, Recife, Brazil

2 Independent Professional, Maceió, Brazil

3 Independent Professional in Physiotherapy, Recife, Brazil

4 Independent Professional in Biology and Mathematics, Recife, Brazil

5 Independent Professional in Production Engineering and Mathematics, Recife, Brazil

*Address all correspondence to: hdorias@gmail.com

References

[1] Werner L, Trindade F, Pereira F, Werner L. Physiology of accommodation and presbyopia. Arquivos Brasileiros de Oftalmologia, 2000, vol. 63, no. 6, p. 487-493. http://dx.doi.org/10.1590/S0004-27492000000600011.

[2] Silva HD, Silva ED, Silva MTD, Dória CaP, Dória CeP. Intraocular forced convection mechanism defect as normal tension glaucoma probable cause. In: GiudiceGLo, editors, Visual Impairment and Blindness - What We Know and What We Have to Know, London, IntechOpen, 2019, p. 120-163. DOI: http://dx.doi.org/10.5772/intechopen.89934.

[3] Silva HD, Dória LCP, Dória CaP, Dória CeP, Silva MCTD, Silva Jr. HD, Silva MTD. Simulation of the Errors of Refraction in the Human Eye. In: Öchsner A, da Silva LFM, Altenbach H, editors. Analysis and Design of Biological Materials and Structures. Advanced Structured Materials book series V. 14. Berlin, Heidelberg: Springer: 2012. p. 185-185. DOI: https://doi.org/10.1007/978-3-642-22131-6_15.

[4] Silva HD, Silva ED, Dória CaP, Silva MTD, Dória CeP. Modelagem do sistema intraocular de convecção forçada. Brazilian Journal of Development. 2019; DOI: 10.34117/bjdv5n7-200.

[5] Silva HD, Silva ED, Silva MTD, Dória CaP, Dória CeP. Analysis of the Disturbances Caused by Intraocular Forced Convection Mechanism Failure. In: Zilfyan A, editors, Difficulties in Cataract Surgery, London, IntechOpen, 2018, p. 45-64. DOI: http//dx.doi.org/10.5772/intechopen.72248.

[6] Simply healthcare. [Internet]. Available from: https://provider.simplyhealthcareplans.com/dam/medpolicies/simply/active/guidelines/gl_pw_c169434.html [Accessed: 2020-12-12].

[7] Crespo RMM , Menéndez CV, Uriarte AMA. GLOSARIO DE OFTALMOLOGIA. Revista Habanera de Ciencias Médicas - on line version, v. 6, n. 2, 2007, ISSN 1729-519X.

[8] IOL Monovision For Cataract Surgery. Henry Ford Medical Group [Internet]. Available from: https://www.henryford.com/services/eye/treatments/cataracts/iol-monovision [Accessed: 2020-11-13].

[9] Heiting G. Dominant eye test: How to find your dominant eye. All About Vision [Internet]. 2020. Available from: https://www.allaboutvision.com/resources/dominant-eye-test.htm.

[10] Silva HD, Dória LCP, Dória CaP, Dória CeP, Silva MCTD, Silva Jr. HD, Silva MTD. Analysis of failure mechanism of forced convection in the cornea of the human eye. In: Öchsner A, da Silva LFM, Altenbach H, editors. Analysis and Design of Biological Materials and Structures. Advanced Structured Materials book series V. 14. Berlin, Heidelberg: Springer: 2012. p. 217-226. https://doi.org/10.1007/978-3-642-31470-4_16.

[11] PierscionekBK,Popiotek-MasajadaA, Kasprzak H. Corneal shape change during accommodation. Eye, 2002 Vol. 15(Pt 6), p. 766-769. DOI: 10.1038/eye.2001.246. https://www.researchgate.net/publication/11533369.

[12] Silva HD, Dória LCP, Dória CaP, Dória CeP, Silva MCTD, Silva Jr. HD, Silva MTD. Simulation of variation of intraocular pressure. In: Öchsner A, da Silva LFM, Altenbach H, editors. Characterization and Development of

Biosystems and Biomaterials. Advanced Structured Materials, 2012; vol 29. Springer, Berlin, Heidelberg. https://doi.org/10.1007/978-3-642-31470-4_18.

[13] Eyeol U.K.. [Internet]. Available from: http://eyeol.co.uk/twb/hydrophilic-iols/foldable-iols/ [Accessed: 2020-12-12].

[14] Silva HD, Dória LCP, Dória CaP, Dória CeP, Silva MCTD, Silva Jr. HD, Silva MTD. Nutrients and metabolic secretions transfer in cornea. Defect and Diffusion Forum, 2011; Vols. 312-315, p. 737-742. http://www.scientific.net/DDF.312-315.737.

[15] Silva HD, Dória LCP, Dória CaP, Dória CeP, Silva MCTD, Silva Jr. HD, Silva MTD. Mass transport mechanism in the retina of the human eye. Defect and Diffusion Forum, 2012; Vols. 326-328, p. 18-23. http://www.scientific.net/DDF.326-328.18.

[16] Silva HD, Dória LCP, Dória CaP, Dória CeP, Silva MCTD, Silva Jr. HD, Silva MTD. Forced Convection Mechanism Failure in the Eye Can Cause Macular Degeneration. Defect and Diffusion Forum, 2013; Vols. 334-335, p. 230-234. https://doi.org/10.4028/www.scientific.net/DDF.334-335.230.

[17] Silva HD, Dória LCP, Dória CaP, Dória CeP, Silva MCTD, Silva Jr. HD, Silva MTD. Forced Convection Mechanism Failure in the Eye Can Cause Cataract. Defect and Diffusion Forum, 2013; Vols. 334-335, p. 225-229. DOI: https://doi.org/10.4028/www.scientific.net/DDF.334-335.225.

[18] Bicas HEA, Jorge AAH. Oftalmologia: fundamentos e aplicações. 1st. Edition São Paulo, SP, Tecmedd editor, 2007, ISBN-10: 8599276182.

[19] Burge J, Rodriguez-Lopez V, Dorronsoro C. Monovision and the Misperception of Motion. Curr Biol., 2019; Vol. 29, p. 2586-2592.e4. DOI: 10.1016/j.cub.2019.06.070. https://www.sciencedirect.com/science/article/pii/S0960982219307973.

[20] Smith CE, Allison RS, Wilkinson F, Wilcox LM. Monovision: Consequences for depth perception from large disparities. Experimental Eye Research, 2018; https://www.researchgate.net/publication/327693427 DOI: 10.1016/j.exer.2018.09.005

[21] Pinhole glasses. Wikipedia,the free encyclopedia. [Internet]. Available from: https://en.wikipedia.org/wiki/Pinhole_glasses [Accessed: 2020-12-12].

Section 3

Visual Quanlity Improvement

Chapter 6

Pseudophakic Presbyopic Corrections

Georgios Labiris and Eirini-Kanella Panagiotopoulou

Abstract

Presbyopia is a prevalent productivity-reducing, age-related visual disorder that results in a progressive near vision impairment. Conventional treatment modalities (ie. presbyopic spectacles or contact lenses) are associated with poor acceptance, productivity loss and negative impact on life quality. However, a variety of surgical methods are available to address presbyopia; among them, multifocal and multifocal toric intraocular lenses (IOLs) and monovision techniques. For the best possible refractive outcomes, the overall management of presbyopic patients is necessary. Specifically, patient selection according to personality and daily activities, topography, aberrometry, astigmatism, pupil and fundus assessment, ophthalmic surface, and premium lens selection should be taken into consideration. Additionally, image-guided surgery could increase the accuracy in multifocal/multifocal toric IOL implantation, and optimize the refractive outcome increasing patient satisfaction. Primary objective of this chapter is to analyze the fundamental preoperative, intraoperative and postoperative management of patients that undergo pseudophakic presbyopic corrections with conventional or digital-marking assisted techniques.

Keywords: presbyopia, cataract surgery, refractive lens exchange, multifocal intraocular lens, monovision, pseudophakic presbyopic correction

1. Introduction

Presbyopia is probably the most prevalent productivity-reducing, age-related visual disorder that results in a progressive impairment of near vision capacity Presbyopia symptoms include blurry vision when targeting at near objects and fatigue when reading, especially in suboptimal lighting conditions. It is common for emmetropic populations above 40 years old. Almost every working person is expected to suffer from reduction of his/her near and intermediate vision capacity due to presbyopia [1, 2]. Taking into consideration the constantly increasing life-expectancy, conservative estimates suggest that by 2050, about 1.8 billion people will experience presbyopia symptoms [3]. Additionally, since computers, tablets, and smart phones have modified heavily working and social norms, presbyopia significantly limits the patient's productivity and reduces life quality [4, 5].

It is a truism that correction of presbyopia is among the most challenging unmet objectives in Ophthalmology. Conventional treatment modalities (ie. presbyopic spectacles or contact lenses) are associated with poor acceptance, productivity loss and significant negative impact on the quality of life [5]. Despite the fact that the lens extraction surgery is the most frequent surgical operation in Medicine, [5, 6] the postoperative loss of accommodation is yet to be adequately addressed. Different surgical approaches for the correction of presbyopia have been developed targeting the cornea and/or the crystalline lens [7]. A variety of technologies have also been introduced, primarily in the ophthalmological lasers and in the intraocular lenses (IOLs) aiming to restore the pre-presbyopic functionality of the human eye [8]. The ultimate goal is a spectacle-free visual capacity that imposes no limits to the social, personal, working needs of each patient [9–12]. As regards pseudophakic presbyopic corrections, the "ideal" IOL should restore the patients' vision without complications or visual compromises at all distances [13]. Premium IOLs, such as multifocal, accommodating and extended-depth-of-focus (EDOF), as well as pseudophakic monovision techniques achieved by monofocal IOL implantation or implantation of a combination of premium IOLs, are some of the available surgical approaches. When presbyopia is combined with astigmatism, multifocal toric IOLs can be used.

However, for the best possible refractive outcomes, solid and up-to-date information on the overall management of presbyopic patients is necessary. In specific, patient selection (according to personality, daily activities, and expectations), astigmatism assessment, topography, aberrometry, pupil assessment, ophthalmic surface, fundus assessment, and premium lens selection should always be taken into consideration before a presbyopic correction. In addition, in case of implantation of multifocal or multifocal toric IOLs, image-guided surgery could increase the accuracy of IOL centration (in multifocal and multifocal toric IOLs) and alignment (in multifocal toric IOLs), and optimize the refractive outcome increasing patient satisfaction.

Primary objective of this chapter is to analyze the fundamental preoperative, intraoperative and postoperative management of patients that undergo pseudophakic presbyopic correction with conventional or digital-marking assisted techniques. In specific, this chapter aims to give an overview of the current IOL technologies for a pseudophakic presbyopic correction, patient selection criteria, benefits and limitations of each IOL technology.

2. Preoperative diagnostic evaluation

Accurate preoperative diagnostic evaluation is necessary for preoperative patient counseling, the selection of the most appropriate IOL type and surgical planning. Preoperative diagnostics are also essential for determining the anatomical success rates of IOL implantation [13].

A preoperative examination for patients intending to undergo a pseudophakic presbyopic correction should include: (i) taking of the medical history, (ii) basic ophthalmological examination, and (iii) additional diagnostic procedures:

2.1 Medical history

2.1.1 General medical history

As in the routine preoperative examination for a typical cataract surgery with implantation of a monofocal IOL, the routine preoperative examination for a pseudophakic presbyopic correction should include taking a detailed history for current or past medical conditions [eg. hypertension, diabetes, ischemic heart disease, pulmonary diseases, benign prostatic hyperplasia (BPH), bleeding disorders, history of herpes libialis or autoimmune diseases, such as rheumatoid arthritis, Hashimoto's thyroiditis, and Sjogren syndrome].

In addition, the surgeon should be aware of the patient's former surgeries and current or prior use of systemic or topical pharmaceutical medications such as anticoagulant, alpha-blocker (tamsulosin) for BPH, steroid or immunosuppressant medication [14].

2.1.2 Ocular history

Glaucoma, former incisional surgery (eg. refractive, retinal, glaucoma, muscle surgery), eye trauma, amblyopia, herpes simplex keratitis, allergic conjunctivitis, uveitis, recurrent corneal erosions and prior or current topical medications should be taken into account.

2.1.3 Family eye history

Family history of eye disorders responsible for blindness or visual impairment (e.g. glaucoma, retinal or corneal disease, etc) should be considered.

2.1.4 Allergies

If the patient is allergic to medications, the type of medication and the exact reaction to that medication should be clarified (rash, anaphylaxis etc).

2.2 Basic ophthalmological examination

2.2.1 Visual acuity assessment

The evaluation of the Uncorrected Distance Visual Acuity (UDVA), Best Corrected Distance Visual Acuity (BCDVA), Uncorrected Near Visual Acuity (UNVA), Best Corrected Near Visual Acuity (BCNVA), Uncorrected Intermediate Visual Acuity (UIVA), Best Corrected Intermediate Visual Acuity (BCIVA) should be included in the ophthalmic examination. The contrast sensitivity should also be evaluated.

2.2.2 Slit lamp examination of the anterior segments of the eye

Eyelids, lacrimal drainage system, cornea, conjunctiva, iris, pupil, anterior chamber, and lens should be evaluated in the first preoperative examination. In detail, certain findings for each anatomical structure should be taken into account and could encourage surgeons to perform some types of presbyopic corrections or discourage them from performing other surgical techniques. In addition, some eye pathologies should be addressed before the surgery.

- *Eyelids:* Eyelid pathology, including ectropion, entropion, and blepharitis, should be addressed before the surgery.

- *Lacrimal drainage system:* The lacrimal drainage system is recommended to be open.

- *Cornea:* Ocular surface and cornea should be evaluated. Ocular surface disease such as dry-eye syndrome, exposure keratitis and meibomian gland dysfunction should be treated preoperatively, since tear-film abnormalities may influence postoperative visual outcomes leading to suboptimal visual quality and performance, regardless of the type of IOL to be implanted. Slit lamp evaluation of corneal endothelium should not be omitted. Corneal dystrophies, such as Fuchs' corneal dystrophy, as well as corneal scars (central or peripheral), pterygium and keratoconus signs should be taken into consideration for the selection of the most appropriate presbyopia correction method.

- *Conjunctiva:* Conjunctival disorders should be assessed, such as conjunctival hyperemia, papillae, hyperplasia of lymphoid follicles, erosions, scarring and symblepharon.

- *Iris:* The pupil size and shape should be evaluated before and after mydriasis. Pupils with an irregular shape could interfere with desired refractive outcome. Inadequate mydriasis is a well-known risk factor associated with numerous intra- or postoperative complications [15]. In addition, anterior and/or posterior synechiae could increase the risk for inadequate mydriasis and intraoperative complications. Finally, iris neovascularization should not be overlooked.

- *Anterior chamber:* The anterior chamber depth (ACD) should be evaluated with slit lamp biomicroscopy. A shallow anterior chamber can be present in hypermetropic eyes with short axial length (AL). However, it might also be caused by an intumescent cataract or other pathological causes. Regardless of the cause, a shallow anterior chamber could increase the difficulty of a lens extraction surgery. Finally, gonioscopy could be performed, if considered necessary, to reveal angle abnormalities like synechiae and neovascularization.

- *Lens:* The cataract type and density should be evaluated in order to predict possible technical difficulties in performing cataract surgery. In addition, the presence of Pseudoexfoliation Syndrome (PEX), which is the most common cause of zonular weakness, should be identified. PEX can be better revealed after pupil dilation. This should be taken into account for the IOL type selection, since it increases the risk of a possible late decentration and misalignment of the IOL, that could influence the visual outcome negatively.

2.2.3 Slit lamp examination of the posterior segments of the eye (under pupil dilation)

- *Optic nerve:* Any abnormality of the optic nerve could influence the surgeon's decision for the IOL type selection.

- *Macula:* The macular anatomy should be assessed. The presence of acquired macular disorders including age-related macular degeneration (ARMD) findings and macular edema, or hereditary macular disorders, such as Stargardt's disease and retinitis pigmentosa, could be considered as relative or absolute contraindications for pseudophakic presbyopic corrections. The evaluation of the appropriateness of a pseudophakic presbyopic correction in the presence of a macular disease should depend on the stability of the disease, the expected progression over time, and the availability and usefulness of its treatment.

- *Rest fundus:* Retinal ischemia, vitreous retinal traction, lattice degeneration, and macular hole should be sought especially in diabetic patients.

2.2.4 Intraocular pressure (IOP) measurement

The measurement of the IOP should be part of the basic ophthalmological examination.

2.3 Additional diagnostic procedures

2.3.1 Automatic refraction

Measurements taken by an automatic kerato-refractometer can be co-evaluated with manifest refraction and corneal topography for the confirmation of the refractive error.

2.3.2 Optical biometry

Optical biometry, which is based on monochromatic light-emitting diodes, [16] including partial coherence interferometry (PCI) [e.g. IOLMaster 500 (Carl Zeiss Meditec AG, Jena, Germany)] and swept source OCT (ss-OCT) [eg. IOLMaster 700 (Carl Zeiss Meditec AG, Jena, Germany), Anterion (Heidelberg Engineering, Heidelberg, Germany)], serves as highly reliable method for AL (in mm), ACD (in mm) and keratometry (in diopters) determination. In comparison with standard keratometry, total keratometry measured with ss-OCT (IOLMaster 700) is a new measurement for the assessment of anterior and posterior corneal curvatures that seems to show higher accuracy in IOL power calculation and better refractive outcomes in eyes with or without previous laser refractive surgery [17–19]. As a result, it has been established as the most common preoperative examination performed to calculate the IOL power. According to the selected technique and patient, the postoperative refractive target is plano, low myopia or low hyperopia [20]. A variety of formulas have been used for the most accurate IOL power calculation. Since it has been found that inaccurate biometry is the most common cause of residual postoperative refractive error, [21] some factors should be taken into account; among them, interocular consistency in AL and K values, appropriate formula for each case, and outliers [22]. Last but not least, preoperatively, the surgeon should check and confirm that the biometry corresponds to the correct patient.

2.3.3 A-scan ultrasound biometry

Although A-scan biometry is less accurate and requires more operator skills to ensure consistent accuracy in comparison with optical biometry, it can be used in presence of dense cataract or corneal edema when the optical biometry cannot take measurements [23]. However, for the optimization of a-scan results, the immersion instead of the applanation (contact) technique could be chosen, since the former has better repeatability and higher accuracy than the latter [24, 25].

2.3.4 Corneal pachymetry

Ultrasonic pachymetry may contribute to the assessment of overall endothelial function in corneas with a diseased endothelium or with borderline low endothelial cell counts, however, corneal central thickness is not correlated with endothelial cell numerical density within the physiological range. Specifically, an increased preoperative thickness might increase the risk for postoperative clinical corneal edema [26].

2.3.5 Scheimpflug tomography/placido-based corneal topography

Scheimpflug tomography or, alternatively, placido-based corneal topography can determine patient's total or anterior-surface corneal astigmatism, respectively, and whether the astigmatism is regular or irregular, or even detect possible keratoconus. The corneal topographic analysis should be compared with optical biometry findings for the best possible accuracy in IOL power and astigmatism calculation, especially if a laser refractive surgery has been preceded.

2.3.6 Aberrometry

The routine preoperative examination should include the determination of the anterior aberration profile looking for elevations of 3rd- and 4th-order aberrations, such as coma and spherical aberrations (SA) [27]. Generally, cornea has an average positive SA of +0.28 μm (positive SA occurs when the peripheral rays entering the eye are focused in front of the central rays) [28]. Among the most common aberrometers are i-Trace aberrometer (Tracey Technologies Corp., Houston, TX), OPD-scan (ARK 10000; Nidek), and Pentacam (Oculus Optikgerate GmbH, Wetzlar, Germany), which calculate total ocular, lens or corneal wavefront aberrations [29, 30].

2.3.7 Pupillometry

Preoperative pupillometry can measure: (i) pupil diameter under photopic (small pupil) and mesopic (wide pupil) lighting conditions, (ii) distance between the pupil center and the visual axis (angle kappa), between the corneal center and the visual axis (angle alpha), and/or between the pupil center and the corneal center, and (iii) distance (spatial shift) from the photopic to the mesopic pupil center (pupil center shift - PCS) [31–33]. Regarding PCS, two types of PCS can be evaluated: (i) measured PCS, which results from the values measured under photopic and mesopic lighting conditions, and (ii) interpolated PCS, which depicts the predicted spatial shift between a photopic pupil of 2 mm to a scotopic pupil of 7 mm, and can contribute to the better comparability of the measurements [34].

2.3.8 Specular microscopy

Endotheliometry, especially in suspicion of endothelial dysfunction/dystrophy, is a very useful examination. The average endothelial cell density (ECD) in patients > 40 years old ranges between about 2500 and 2700 cells/mm^2 [35]. A central ECD decline of less than 1000 cells/mm^2 preoperatively, and 400 to 700 cells/mm^2 postoperatively might cause significant postoperative endothelial cell impairment and corneal edema. The hexagonality should also be assessed [36–38].

2.3.9 Macula and ONH OCT - OCTA

Since good macular and optic nerve function are necessary for a premium pseudophakic presbyopic correction, many surgeons perform an optical coherence tomography (OCT), or even an OCT angiography (OCTA), of the macula and optic nerve head (ONH) to confirm normal macular and optic nerve anatomy and microcirculation. Macular degeneration, subtle epiretinal membranes, early stages of macular hole or posterior vitreous separation with vitreal macular traction, but also glaucoma or vascular abnormalities in various optic neuropathies can be revealed.

2.3.10 Anterior segment OCT (AS-OCT)

The application of AS-OCT during the preoperative planning for cataract surgery could be useful in the accurate prediction of postoperative ACD and postoperative IOL position [39, 40].

2.3.11 B-mode ultrasonography

This examination could be performed to detect the posterior segment disorders, especially in suspicion of retinal detachment, vitreous opacity or posterior segment tumor, especially when the fundoscopy is impossible due to mature cataract.

2.3.12 Image-guided systems – preoperative units

The size and the location of main and sideport incisions, the size and diameter of capsulorrhexis, the centration of the capsulorrhexis, as well as the alignment axis in case of toric or multifocal toric IOLs are predetermined in the preoperative examination with the measurement module of image-guided lens extraction surgery systems [41].

3. Surgical procedures – IOL types

The two most widely used methods for pseudophakic presbyopic correction are the monovision technique through bilateral implantation of monofocal IOLs and the bilateral implantation of multifocal IOLs [8].

3.1 Monovision techniques with bilateral monofocal IOL implantation

Pseudophakic, or IOL, monovision, which was first described by Boerner and Thrasher in 1984, [42] still remains the most common surgical management of presbyopia for cataract patients with good spectacle independence and high patient satisfaction [43, 44]. The 2016 clinical survey of the European Society of Cataract and Refractive Surgery (ESCRS) reported that 43% of cataract procedures are targeted for monovision or mini-monovision [45].

In traditional pseudophakic monovision, monofocal IOLs are implanted in both eyes. However, the recessive eye is intentionally defocused for myopia [8, 10, 12]. Myopic defocus of the recessive eye ranges from over 2 diopters (D) to less than 1 D (mini or micro monovision) [8, 10, 46]. In bilateral myopic monovision, the dominant eye defocus is targeted to -0.50 D, while the recessive one to -1.25 D [47]. However, recently, the crossed monovision has been suggested for high myopic cataract patients, which is to correct the dominant eye for near vision and the non-dominant eye for distance vision [8].

3.1.1 Patient selection

A careful patient selection with a specific determination of the inclusion and exclusion criteria is of paramount importance for an optimal refractive outcome and the highest possible patient satisfaction in case of pseudophakic monovision with bilateral monofocal IOL implantation.

Inclusion criteria: The most frequent inclusion criterion was the desire for spectacle independence [48]. One of the most important prerequisites for monovision success is the weak ocular dominance [49, 50].

Exclusion criteria: Several exclusion criteria have been reported in the literature. Some of them are the following:

- *Severe ocular diseases:* Patients with pathology of the optic nerve (eg. glaucoma or other optic neuropathies), macular or retinal pathology, corneal pathology or severe opacification of the rest refractive media other than cataract, previous history of ocular inflammation or surgery, amblyopia and other ocular pathology affecting visual performance are commonly excluded from monovision techniques [48], since the aforementioned diseases are believed to have suboptimal effect on visual rehabilitation [49].

- *Corneal astigmatism:* Patients with corneal astigmatism of ≥ 1.00 D, but also of ≥ 1.50 D or even ≥ 2.00 D are commonly excluded from monovision surgical methods with monofocal IOLs [48]. In fact, patients with high degree of corneal astigmatism do not benefit from monovision because their monocular and binocular UVA remains suboptimal. However, the implantation of toric IOLs could be considered. Moreover, patient satisfaction is related to the distance UVA of the dominant eye. Therefore, the correction of corneal astigmatism to less than 1.00 D is highly recommended [49].

- *Strong ocular dominance:* In patients with strong ocular dominance, the artificial anisometropia of monovision causes insufficient blur suppression and leads to reduction in visual performance [48, 50].

- *History of strabismus and abnormal ocular position (exophoria or esophoria):* Patients with a history of strabismus should be informed that monovision might lead to a recurrence of previous strabismus or asthenopic symptoms, and patients with a significant exophoria or esophoria should be informed that monovision might cause strabismus. Nevertheless, if patients wish to proceed to monovision, small levels of anisometropia, such as 1.25 to 1.50 D should be chosen to minimize the chance of strabismus [48, 51].

- *Age, lifestyle, work:* Patients younger than 60 years undergoing pseudophakic monovision seem to have lower postoperative satisfaction in comparison to patients older than 60 years. Some reasons for dissatisfaction are the higher rates of spectacle independence, asthenopia and difficulty mainly in near vision. This likely reflects the different age-related lifestyle activities between younger and older patients [52]. As a result, age lower than 60 years could be considered as an exclusion criterion, especially if it is combined with work requiring precise near vision. Pseudophakic monovision seems to be more beneficial for people older than 60 years [49, 52].

- *Nighttime driving, work under low illuminance:* In cases of weak ocular dominance, when the optical target appears highly contrasted with the background under mesopic lighting conditions, blur suppression does not function sufficiently. Therefore, pseudophakic monovision should be avoided in patients whose work requires precise vision under low illuminance levels or driving at night [52].

- *Inability to understand the concept of monovision design* [53]

In conclusion, regardless of the exclusion criteria, it is suggested that the procedure and possible outcomes of pseudophakic monovision, when selected, should be thoroughly explained to patients in order the best possible visual outcome and patient satisfaction to be achieved.

3.1.2 Side effects of monovision technique

Although monovision is the most common surgical management of presbyopia for cataract patients with millions of people having monovision corrections, some important drawbacks of this method should be described.

First, although monovision is related with significant satisfaction, the highest percentages of satisfied patients have been found in age older than 70 years, while patients younger than 60 years have the highest percentages of dissatisfaction caused mainly by asthenopia and spectacle dependence [52].

Secondly, it has been reported that anisometropia and blur differences cause a motion illusion that leads to a significant misperception of the distance and three-dimensional direction of moving objects, since the blurred and sharp images are processed at different speeds. This phenomenon has a clinical impact on driving behavior, since these millisecond differences in processing speed could lead, for instance, to the misperception of the distance of cyclists by the width of a narrow street lane [54].

Finally, depth perception and distance stereopsis, especially for large disparities, may be compromised increasing the difficulty in navigation through the environment, obstacle avoidance, and stair walking. Reduction of distance stereopsis leads to a decrease in stability during locomotion, as well, increasing the risk factor for falls and hip fractures in aged population [55]. Near stereopsis is also reduced, although it remains within the normal range [52].

3.2 Multifocal IOLs

Multifocal IOLs have been designed to provide spectacle independence at near, intermediate, and distance vision tasks. The first concept of a truly multifocal IOL was conceived in 1983 by Hoffer, [56] and the first bifocal IOL implantation was performed by Pearce in 1986 [57]. Since then, many modifications and improvements in multifocal IOL concept have been made [58].

Before the analysis of the pre-, intra- and postoperative management of patients implanted with mIOLs, a brief description of the optical design and properties of mIOLs is required.

3.2.1 Optical design and properties of mIOLs

Two optical phenomena can be utilized to create multifocal optics: refraction and diffraction.

3.2.1.1 Fully refractive IOLs

Fully refractive multifocal IOLs direct light at different focal points using concentric zones of varying dioptric power within the optic. The optical power depends on the local surface curvature, with regions of differing curvatures achieving different powers within the lens. These IOLs are also called *multizonal refractive IOLs* (**Figure 1**) [59]. The central circular zone has a power corresponding to distance vision. The surrounding annular zones alternate between powers corresponding to near and distance to achieve the multifocal effect [60]. As the pupillary size changes, the number of zones that are utilized varies, and, subsequently, the relative proportion of light directed to the distant, near and/or intermediate focal points changes as well [59]. Thus, image quality can fluctuate depending on pupil size [61, 62].

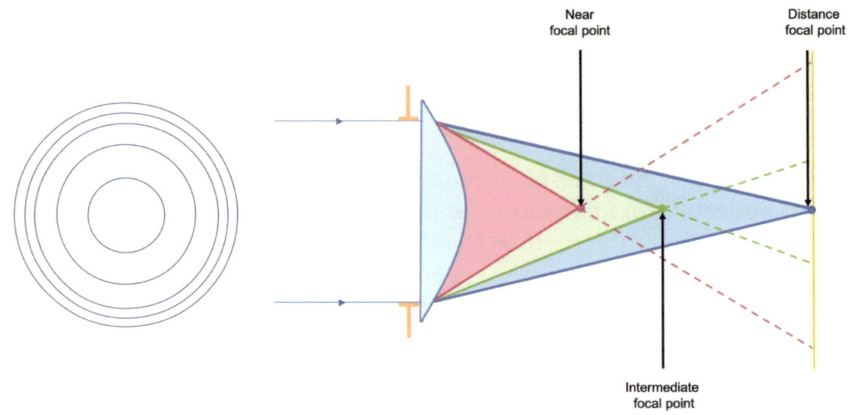

Figure 1.
Refractive IOL design – focal points.

3.2.1.2 Diffractive IOLs

To create multifocality, diffractive multifocal IOLs use the optical phenomenon of diffraction and take advantage of the wave nature of light by selectively delaying the optical path in selected areas and slightly changing its direction when encountering an edge or discontinuity [59–62]. Typical diffractive multifocal IOLs consist of concentric annular zones in their anterior or posterior surface that constitute an asymmetrical zone plate, also referred as "diffractive kinoform" (**Figure 2**) [63]. The spacing between the zones gets progressively smaller from the center towards the edge of the IOL. Abrupt steps appear at the junction of each zone. These microscopic steps on the diffractive surface of the IOL with height of a few microns have a specific phase delay. The area of each zone determines the add power of the IOL and the maximum height of the steps determines the relative amount of light energy distributed on each focus [60, 61]. In fact, the heights of each step are chosen in such a way that approximately 40 – 40.5% of the incident light contributes to the add portion, 40 – 40.5% of the incident light contributes to the distance portion and the remaining light goes into other diffractive foci. Alternative step heights can be chosen to shift more energy to either the distance or near focus. Therefore, the diffractive element of these IOLs enables the splitting of the incoming light into two or three foci for bifocal and trifocal IOLs, respectively [60, 61].

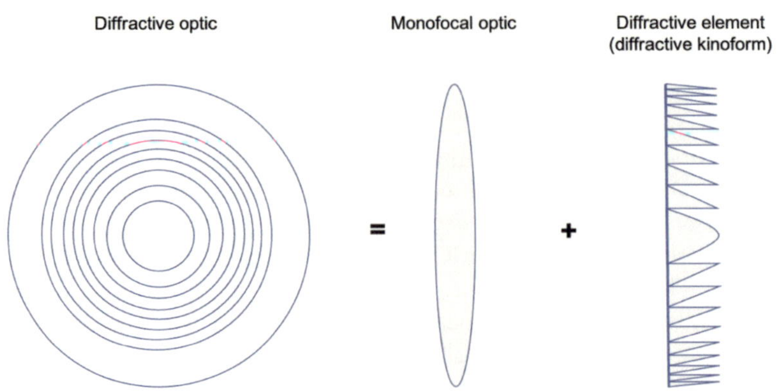

Figure 2.
Diffractive IOL design.

A further division of diffractive multifocal IOLs is based on *apodization*, which is the gradual decrease of the height of the steps from the center of the optic to its periphery [61]. Thus, diffractive IOLs can be classified into those with apodized and those with non-apodized diffractive optics (**Figure 3**).

3.2.1.2.1 Apodized diffractive IOLs

The characteristic of apodized diffractive IOLs is a decrease in height from the taller central to the shorter peripheral steps of the optic [59]. The lower steps of the periphery send more energy to the far and less to the near focal point. On the contrary, the higher central steps send equal energy to distance and near [64]. The clinical significance of this phenomenon is shown by the fact that the larger pupil diameter in scotopic light conditions, when only the distance vision is utilized, allows more energy to be directed to the distance focal point, while the smaller pupil diameter in photopic conditions, when both distance and near vision are utilized, allows energy to be directed equally to distance and near (**Figure 4**) [60, 64]. Additionally, apodized diffractive IOLs produce fewer optic phenomena (eg. glare, halos etc) than non-apodized IOL during distance vision through a large pupil [59].

Some characteristic apodized diffractive IOL models are the following:

- AcrySof IQ ReSTOR SN6AD1 (Alcon Laboratories, Inc., Fort Worth, TX, USA): a single-piece, bifocal, symmetric biconvex IOL with an aspheric diffractive, apodized, anterior surface (+3.0 D near add power at the IOL plane) [65].

- AcrySof IQ ReSTOR SN6AD2 [SV25T0] (Alcon Laboratories, Inc., Fort Worth, TX, USA): a single-piece, apodized, diffractive aspheric bifocal IOL with a central refractive zone (*hybrid IOL*) (+2.5 D near add power at the IOL plane) [66].

- FineVision IOL (PhysIOL, Liege, Belgium): a single-piece, apodized, diffractive trifocal (+1.75 D intermediate and +3.5 D near add power at the IOL plane), aspheric IOL (aspheric posterior surface and diffractive anterior surface) [67].

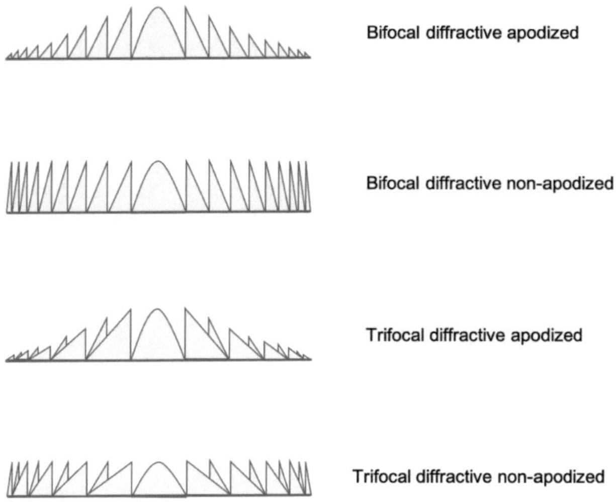

Figure 3.
Examples of diffractive multifocal IOL designs.

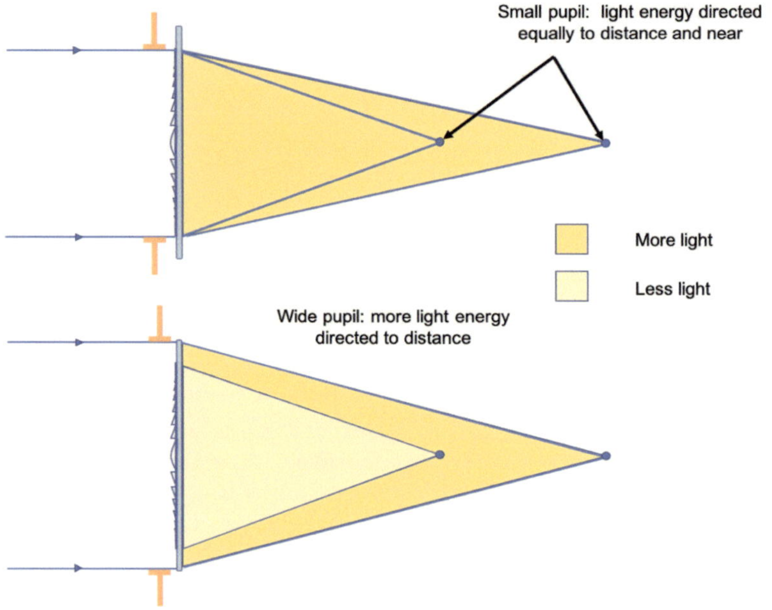

Figure 4.
Light distribution in photopic (A) and mesopic-scotopic (B) light conditions in diffractive apodized IOL designs. (A) The small pupil diameter in photopic conditions, when both distance and near vision are utilized, allows light energy to be directed equally to distance and near. (B) The wide pupil diameter in low light conditions, when only the distance vision is utilized, allows more energy to be directed to the distance focal point.

3.2.1.2.2 Non-apodized diffractive IOLs

In contrast to the apodized IOLs, the diffractive steps of non-apodized diffractive IOLs have uniform height from the center to the periphery. Therefore, these IOLs can distribute the light rays to near and distant focal points in constant proportions, irrespectively of the pupillary size [61, 68]. However, they sacrifice some intermediate vision, and may produce more photic phenomena than apodized diffractive IOLs [62].

Some characteristic non-apodized diffractive IOL models are the following:

- AcrySof IQ PanOptix (Alcon Laboratories, Inc., Fort Worth, TX, USA): a single-piece diffractive, non-apodized, aspheric (spherical posterior surface and aspheric anterior surface with a diffractive surface on the central 4.5 mm), trifocal IOL (+2.17 D intermediate and +3.25 D near add power at the IOL plane) [69].

- TECNIS multifocal IOL (AMO, Santa Ana, CA): a single-piece diffractive, non-apodized, aspheric (aspheric anterior surface, full-diffractive posterior surface), bifocal IOL (ZMB00: +4.00 D / ZLB00: +3.25 D / ZKB00: +2.75 D add power) [70].

- AT LISA 809 IOL (Carl Zeiss Meditec AG, Jena, Germany): a single-piece diffractive, non-apodized, aspheric bifocal (+3.75 D near add power at the IOL plane), biconvex IOL [71].

- AT LISA TRI 839MP (IOL (Carl Zeiss Meditec AG, Jena, Germany): a single-piece diffractive, non-apodized, aspheric trifocal IOL (+1.66 D intermediate and +3.33 D near add power at the IOL plane) [72].

3.2.2 Preoperative counseling, preoperative examination and patient selection

Preoperative counseling and patient selection play a pivotal role in the success of pseudophakic presbyopic correction with implantation of mIOLs. It is well known that patients wishing to undergo presbyopic correction have high expectations for their visual and refractive outcome. Thus, it is common that some patients with a visual acuity of 0.0 logMAR are not fully satisfied usually due to photic phenomena at scotopic or mesopic light conditions (e.g. during nighttime driving) and difficulty in reading of very small letters or small letters under lower lighting levels. Some possible reasons of dissatisfaction are potential optical aberrations, residual astigmatism, large pupil and slow or no neuroadaptation [13]. For this reason, a good counseling and a thorough preoperative examination should be an integral part of the preoperative patient management for the best possible patient selection and determination of patient's expectations.

3.2.2.1 Clinical factors/exclusion criteria, contraindications

Before the discussion between patient and surgeon for an eventual pseudophakic presbyopic correction with implantation of a mIOL, a detailed patient history should be taken and a first general ophthalmologic examination (VA, slit-lamp biomicroscopy, IOP measurement) should be performed, which might reveal some clinical parameters that could rule out this type of surgery; among them, significant preexisting ocular pathology that could reduce the postoperative visual outcome, severe untreated dry eye disease, Fuch's endothelial dystrophy or other corneal dystrophies, keratoconus, corneal scars, macular degeneration, diabetic retinopathy or other retinal disease, advanced glaucoma or other optic nerve diseases, and amblyopia. In addition, mIOLs should be avoided in patients with pupillary abnormalities such as corectopia and colobomas, as well as in patients with phacodonesis zonular dialysis or pseudoexfoliation due to the high risk of IOL decentration [61, 64].

3.2.2.2 Patient factors/preoperative counseling

The history taking and the general ophthalmologic examination should be followed by a detailed preoperative counseling. As part of the counseling, each patient should be warned about the risks of the lens extraction surgery, but also for the specific risks of the implantation of a mIOL. The selection of both the proper patient and the proper mIOL results in high patient satisfaction rates. Specifically, the following aspects should be discussed:

The determination of each patient's personality type, lifestyle, hobbies, needs, occupation, and expectations should not be omitted.

- *Personality:* Surgeons should be cautious about selecting patients with a type A personality. Specifically, patients with neurotic personality traits are less likely to be satisfied with the postoperative outcome in comparison with patients whose dominant personality trait is conscientiousness and agreeableness [73]. Additionally, the personality characteristics of compulsive checking, orderliness, competence, and dutifulness have found to be related to subjective disturbance by glare and halos [74].

- *Lifestyle, hobbies, needs:* Patients who read a lot may benefit more from a mIOL that provides better near vision, while patients who use a computer may benefit more from a mIOL that provides better intermediate vision. Trifocal IOLs would be a good solution for patients that need both near and intermediate vision [64]. In addition, patients who drive at night for long periods of time should not be considered as good mIOL candidates.

- *Occupation:* Patients with high occupational visual demands such as pilots and commercial (public service vehicle, taxi, or truck) drivers should be avoided from mIOL implantation [13, 61].

- *Expectations*: Hypercritical patients with unrealistic expectations are not suitable candidates for mIOL implant. For instance, people whose main concern is the sharpest clearest vision and who do not mind wearing near glasses even when reading very small letters or under low lighting conditions, should be ruled out from insertion of mIOLs.

The surgeon should never promise full spectacle independence, but they should explain to patients that there is a good chance that they will not need glasses for the majority of their activities of daily living and that no perfect IOL to simulate their pre-presbyopic continuous vision exists yet [61]. However, spectacles may be needed under highly demanding conditions or during reading under low lighting conditions. Additionally, patients should be counselled about the optimal level and direction of light for easier reading. Finally, patients should be counselled about adverse events including halo, glare, reduced contrast sensitivity as well as discussing neuroadaptation in greater detail [75]. If patients are able to understand all benefits and risks of mIOLs, they could be good candidates to continue the preoperative examination for a potential pseudophakic presbyopic correction with mIOL implantation.

3.2.2.3 Preoperative examination and patient selection

Some significant parameters that should be taken into account during *preoperative examination* for the patient selection for mIOL implantation and, then, for the selection of the appropriate type and power of the IOL are the following:

- *Optical biometry:* Careful biometry is crucial to accurate IOL power calculation and astigmatism management, since inaccurate biometry is the most common cause of residual refractive error postoperatively [76]. Third generation formulas such as the Holladay [77], SRK/T [78] and Hoffer Q [79] provide good outcomes for patients with average AL (22 – 25 mm) and keratometry. In cases of short eyes (AL < 22 mm) with a shallow ACD (< 2.40 mm), formulas that take preoperative ACD into account, such as Haigis, or alternatively Hoffer Q, could be used [80–82]. When dealing with long eyes (AL > 25–26 mm), SRK/T (with optimized constants), is still an accurate solution [83]. Haigis (with optimized constants) is accurate especially for eyes with AL < 30 mm [84]. Finally, new formulas such as Barrett Universal II and Olsen provide good results in long eyes [82, 85].

- *Dense cataract:* In case of dense cataracts when optical biometry measurements have low accuracy, the repetition of measurements could increase the accuracy in IOL power calculation. When no measurements can be taken, A-scan ultrasound biometry can be used. However, since the accuracy of this method is lower than the accuracy of optical biometry, [86–88] and taking into account that even a residual refractive error of 0.50 D, especially in mIOL implantation, can reduce the vision quality and increase photic phenomena, [89–91] the surgeon should be cautious with the choice of the mIOL or even with the decision for a possible non-mIOL pseudophakic presbyopic correction when an ultrasound biometry is used for the IOL power calculation. The surgeon should discuss with the patient the risks caused by the measurement inaccuracy, and may choose an alternative surgical solution according to patient's visual needs and lifestyle.

- *Corneal astigmatism:* Patients undergoing multifocal IOL implantation may not tolerate residual astigmatism of > 1 D or even 0.75 D according to some studies, and a toric multifocal IOL may be required in such cases [92]. For the best possible calculation of the corneal astigmatism, the performance of more than one keratometry technologies is suggested, since no perfect method is available [13]. Ideally, rotary prism technology (auto-keratorefractometers), PCI, corneal Scheimpflug tomography (which also takes into account posterior corneal astigmatism) or Placido-based corneal topography, and keratometry taken by image-guided systems for lens extraction surgery could be used [16]. In case of agreement in corneal cylinder power and axis among the utilized technologies, the surgeon can safely choose the appropriate common cylinder power of the toric IOL and the alignment axis. If the different methods of measuring corneal cylinder produce inconsistent results, the treatment of the ocular surface should be considered and the measurements should be repeated. In addition, the proper patient positioning should be confirmed [93]. Online calculators are also available for the toric/multifocal toric IOL power calculation with very good results because most of them take IOL power and posterior corneal astigmatism into account [94].

- *Pupillary size:* Pupil size, but also pupil position in relation to the near and distance zones of the lens, seem to affect the optical performance of the implanted mIOLs in terms of VA, optical aberration, diffraction, and retinal luminance. Patients with wide pupils in scotopic light conditions who were implanted with mIOLs have a higher risk of poor postoperative contrast sensitivity under mesopic illuminance levels and optical phenomena such as glare, halos, and starbursts [95]. In fact, large pupil size is one of the most common causes of dissatisfaction and photic phenomena in patients with mIOLs [96–98]. Therefore, the pupillary size under photopic and mesopic light conditions before mydriasis must be determined preoperatively to minimize subjective postoperative side effects [95]. Everyday clinical practice has shown that a mesopic pupil size smaller than 5 mm can minimize photic phenomena. In case of pupil size larger than 5 mm, the surgeon should discuss with the patient the risks for dysphotopic phenomena and decide whether to proceed with the multifocal IOL implantation or not depending on the patient's visual needs and lifestyle. An alternative surgical solution could be proposed if multifocal IOLs are excluded. Nevertheless, in all cases regardless of the pupil size, patients should be informed about the possibility of appearance of some optical phenomena which, however, may be reduced with time through the process of neuroadaptation [99].

- *Visual axis, angle kappa:* In pseudophakic presbyopic corrections with implantation of mIOLs, the angle kappa (misalignment between the visual and pupillary axis) [100] should be taken into consideration, especially for hyperopic patients with a large angle kappa [101, 102]. It has been found that large angle kappa is correlated with more glare and halos after implantation of mIOLs [86, 103]. This happens because when decentration of mIOLs is present (intraoperatively or postoperatively), which is more common in eyes with large angle kappa, the light rays pass through a multifocal ring instead of the central optic zone, resulting in glare and halos [104]. Decentration higher than 0.75 mm irrespectively of IOL design has shown both far and near visual function deterioration [96, 105]. Clinical practice and research has shown that inclusion of patients with an angle kappa and angle alpha < 0.5 mm, ideally < 0.3 mm, (primarily in vertical and secondarily in horizontal axis in the Cartesian coordinates plot) both in mesopic and photopic conditions of illumination can minimize the risk for mIOL decentration and postoperative photic phenomena [103]. On the other hand, when angle kappa and angle alpha are > 0.5 mm, multifocal IOLs should be avoided, and monofocal IOLs for binocular distance vision or monovision could be chosen [106].

- *Pupil center shift (PCS):* It has been found that not only the photopic kappa angle, but also the PCS is associated with dysphotopsia after mIOL implantation [102]. In case of patients having a PCS higher than 0.4 mm, surgeons should decide whether the optical zone of mIOL should be centered on the photopic or mesopic/scotopic pupil center. In fact, when interpolated (from photopic 2 mm to scotopic 7 mm pupil) PCS is higher than 0.7 mm, the implantation of mIOLs should be avoided and other types of IOLs should be preferred [34].

- *Aberrations – ocular scattering:* Although aberrations, such as comma, SA or first order astigmatism, contribute to the enlargement of the depth of focus, they can also result in a decrease in contrast sensitivity and quality of vision. For instance, it has been found that anterior corneal coma values higher than 0.32 or 0.33 mm may create intolerable photic phenomena when a diffractive mIOL is implanted, thus contraindication of mIOL implantation has been suggested in higher coma values [13, 107, 108]. Additionally, since angle kappa [109] and PCS [110] can influence ocular aberrations, they should also be co-evaluated with ocular aberrations in order to provide patients with the best possible vision quality. Apart from aberrations, ocular scattering may have an impact on the quality of retinal image, which may be overestimated when only aberrations are taken into account. Therefore, measurement of both aberrations and ocular scattering could contribute to a more accurate assessment of the visual and optical quality [111].

- *Dry eye disease:* Since dry eye disease and cataract are very common in the elderly population, but also the ocular surface and tear film play a significant role in the quality of vision, dry eye disease treatment should be considered as an integral part of the pre- and postoperative patient's management. It is well known that dry eye may reduce the vision quality after mIOL implantation [112]. Additionally, it has been observed that cataract surgery is also responsible for causing dry eye disease or aggravating existing dry eye symptoms [113, 114]. Therefore, artificial tears and eyelid hygiene, but also cyclosporine or autologous platelet-rich plasma (PRP) in more severe cases, should be used pre- and/or postoperatively [112, 115, 116].

- *Previous corneal refractive surgery:* Particular attention should be given to patients who have undergone a prior corneal refractive surgery and are considering a pseudophakic presbyopic correction with mIOL implantation.

    - It is assumed that corneas which have undergone a refractive surgery such as laser in situ keratomileusis (LASIK), photorefractive keratectomy (PRK) or radial keratotomy (RK), have been rendered multifocal and show many aberrations by the laser procedure. As a result, it also assumed that the implantation of a mIOL would further deteriorate the visual function.

- An additional difficulty is the inaccuracy in IOL power calculation that comes from the inaccuracy in the determination of the total corneal refractive power, [64, 117] and the inaccuracy in the estimation of the effective lens position by various IOL power calculation formulas when post-laser corneal powers are used [64, 118].

- Patients having corneas with irregular astigmatism, or more than 1 micron of higher corneal aberrations (HOA), especially if they are caused by high levels of coma, are not good candidates for mIOLs [64]. In addition, eyes with a large pupil (> 4 mm) have more possibilities to appear photic phenomena caused by existing aberrations in comparison with eyes with a small pupil (< 4 mm). As a result, a poorer visual quality under mesopic or glare conditions may occur [119].

- Although mIOLs are usually well tolerated and effective after corneal refractive surgery, refractive surprises can be common, especially in patients with myopia greater than 6.0 D or in those that have undergone LASIK [120, 121]. To increase the refractive predictability and reduce the risk of a suboptimal refractive outcome, the precise IOL power calculation is of paramount importance. Since keratometers are unable to measure accurately K values of the central post-laser cornea and the outer and inner corneal surfaces may change unpredictably after corneal refractive surgeries, a variety of IOL power calculation methods have been suggested [64]. The most accurate method is the *clinical history method*. To apply this method and calculate the central corneal power, the refractive error (spherical equivalent) and the K values prior to the keratorefractive surgery as well as the stable refractive error after the surgery must be available [122, 123]. Apart from the numerous methods and formulas that are available, some online calculators can also be used complementarily for the IOL power calculation [124–126].

- In general, patients that had a previous keratorefractive surgery and want to have an additional pseudophakic presbyopic correction with mIOLs have high expectations for spectacle-free good vision [127]. However, they should always be informed for the possibility of inaccurate measurements, residual refractive error, hyperopic shift, and/or aberrations resulting in photic phenomena especially in mesopic light conditions [128]. Additionally, the surgeon should explain to patients that there is a possibility that they will need to use a miotic agent postoperatively, especially in mesopic and scotopic light conditions, in case of photic phenomena, [129] and that an additional corneal refractive surgery or even a further surgery for exchanging the mIOL may be needed in the future [130]. Ideally, if the corneal surface is irregular with corneal aberrations and a second laser treatment is necessary to correct this irregularity, such a treatment should be better performed prior to the implantation of the mIOL [130].

3.2.3 Surgical technique

Phacoemulsification is the gold standard technique for cataract surgery and refractive lens exchange. Since mIOL implantation requires high precision and various factors should be taken into consideration, in addition to the common ones for the conventional cataract surgery with monofocal IOL implantation, a variety of parameters for the conventional non-image-guided, but also for an image-guided surgical technique, will be discussed in the text below.

For the best possible refractive outcome during mIOL implantation surgery, the following practices are suggested:

3.2.3.1 Conventional non-image-guided surgical technique

- Topical anesthesia and mydriatic drops are instilled before the operation.

- Periorbital skin, eyelids, and the conjunctival sac are prepared with a solution of iodine povidone.

- The surgical technique is performed using a standard technique of sutureless (commonly 2.2-mm) cataract surgery.

- Intracameral anesthesia and potentially intracameral mydriatics are injected.

- Capsulorrhexis should have a diameter between 4.50 to 5.00 mm. Although a diameter larger than 5.00 mm also is recommended to facilitate nuclear and cortical removal, this increases the risk of postoperative optical phenomena caused by the involvement of more concentric rings when the light rays pass through the IOL's optic. Opacification of the remaining anterior capsule can reduce optical phenomena even in eyes with a pupil diameter larger than 5.00 mm (**Figure 5**).

- Another parameter that should be taken into account, especially in eyes with a large angle kappa, is the centration of capsulorrhexis. The capsulorrhexis is suggested to be centered around the microscope light reflection on the anterior capsule (patients' visual axis) rather than around the pupillary axis [131]. However, in the case of a mature cataract where the patient fails to fixate on the microscope light, but also on the lights of the biometry device during the preoperative examination, the implantation of a mIOL should be avoided, since the risk for a decentered implantation is very high. The centration on the pupil center or on the geometric center of the cornea is not considered as a safe alternative solution.

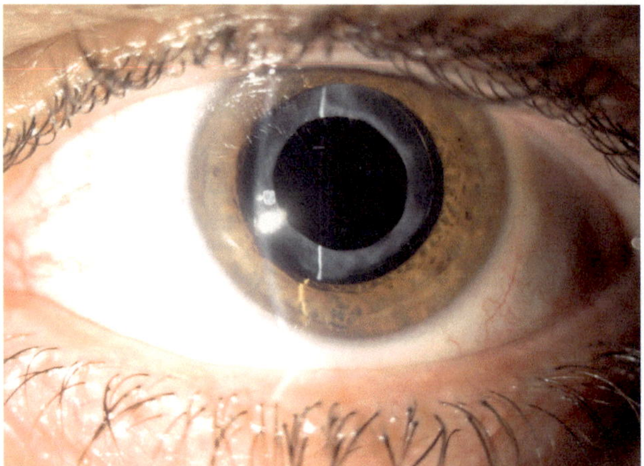

Figure 5.
Anterior capsule opacification following multifocal intraocular lens implantation: the opacification of the remaining anterior capsule contributes in the reduction of potential optical phenomena.

- The nucleus is aspirated with or without ultrasound phacoemulsification energy according to the hardness of the crystalline lens, and residual cortex removal and posterior capsule polishing are performed using commonly bimanual irrigation/aspiration.

- The mIOL is always inserted into the capsular bag through the main incision. The IOL should be injected directly in the capsular bag in order a possibly traumatic surgical manoeuvre to be avoided. For this reason, adequate dilation and an adequate capsulorrhexis of about 4.50 to 5.00 mm is necessary.

- For the optimal mIOL centration and the minimization of photic phenomena, especially for eyes with a large angle kappa, the mIOL is suggested to be decentered towards the visual axis, namely to be gently moved so as the microscope light reflex to fall within the central ring of the multifocal pattern [102]. This is an easy intraoperative manipulation that can effectively result in the desired centration on the visual axis. The centration of diffractive mIOLs on the visual axis is critical to their optimal performance. However, refractive mIOLs are also suggested to be centered on the visual axis because severe cases of decentration can increase the lens' effective power and induce astigmatism and dysphotopsia.

- Additionally, since, normally, the visual axis is nasal to the optical center (the geometric center of the cornea, crystalline lens, and bag after nuclear and cortical removal), positioning the haptics of especially diffractive, but also refractive, IOLs at the 12 and 6 o'clock position may facilitate the desirable nasal displacement of the IOL optic. On the other hand, positioning the IOL haptics horizontally leads to the return of IOL to the geometrically horizontal center [131].

- To stabilize the mIOL centered on the visual axis during the first postoperative days, in contrast to the literature, the authors suggest that a minimal amount of cohesive ophthalmic viscosurgical device (OVD) could be left in the capsular bag without increasing the risk for elevation of the postoperative IOP [132].

- Since mIOL patients usually benefit from having a small pupil, eyes with a small pupil after the instillation of mydriatics before the cataract surgery should be managed with special caution in order the pupil to remain functionally and morphologically intact, as in its preoperative status. Therefore, it is strongly recommended to cataract refractive surgeons to avoid surgical maneuvers such as synechiolysis, pupil stretching, iris cutting [133] and the use of mechanical devices such as iris hooks and pupil expansion rings (e.g. Malyugin ring etc.) because of the high risk of intraoperative disruption of the pupillary sphincter and postoperative pupil enlargement [134]. Thus, intracameral administration of mydriatic agent, combined intracameral use of mydriatic agent and local anesthetic or the injection of OVD into the anterior chamber (viscomydriasis) should be preferred for the pupil dilation [134]. For an experienced refractive cataract surgeon, a possible threshold of pupil size for a successful phacoemulsification ranges between 4.5 and 5.0 mm [134, 135]. In smaller pupils which cannot be dilated pharmacologically or with OVD use, the surgeon should weigh the benefits and the risks of the pupil dilation with surgical maneuvres and mechanical devices and should consider the implantation of a non-mIOL.

- Videorecording of every surgery is suggested for refractive cataract surgeons and, generally, for ophthalmic surgeons in order to review their surgeries, criticize their technique, find mistakes that should have been avoided, explain unexpected outcomes and improve their surgical skills [136].

3.2.3.2 Image-guided surgery

Although the experience and the surgical skills of the refractive cataract surgeon play the most significant role in the final refractive outcome, image-guided lens extraction surgery, which has been recently introduced in phacoemulsification, can increase the surgical accuracy, decrease the risk of complications such as postoperative astigmatism, IOL decentration and photopic phenomena and improve the patient's quality of vision [41].

Image-guided systems such as Verion Digital Marker (Alcon Laboratories, Inc., Fort Worth, TX, USA) [137] and Zeiss Callisto Eye (Carl Zeiss AG, Dublin, CA) [138] are commonly used for the implantation of multifocal toric IOLs. However, since the high accuracy is also necessary during the implantation of multifocal non-toric IOLs for main and sideport incisions, the centration and the diameter of capsulorrhexis, as well as for the centration of the mIOL implantation, the authors suggest that digital image-guidance also during the implantation of multifocal non-toric IOLs could optimize the surgical accuracy and predictability, minimize the risk of complications, and maximize the refractive outcome. **Figure 6** presents the basic steps of lens extraction surgery (a. sideport incisions, b. main incision, c. capsulorrhexis, d. IOL centration, e. finalization) using the Verion image-guided system during the implantation of a multifocal non-toric IOL.

3.2.4 Complications

Implantation of mIOLs provide patients with a good visual acuity at more than one focal point depending on mIOL design. Patient satisfaction levels after mIOL implantation are high. However, the same characteristics that offer refractive correction at all distances can result in adverse effects at the same time [98].

For instance, light distribution mechanisms split the light to two or three focal points. As a result, less amount of light from each focal point reaches the retina worsening the contrast sensitivity, especially in mesopic light conditions [98, 139]. Therefore, two or three distinct images are produced, one sharp on focus and one blurred out of focus. The light of the latter image reduces the detectability of the on-focus image, resulting in the lower contrast sensitivity, however within the normal range of age-matched phakic individuals, and in the creation of dysphotopic phenomena such as halos [139–141]. These phenomena commonly diminish over time through the process of neuroadaptation.

The most common reason for patient dissatisfaction is *blurred vision* (approximately in 95% of the dissatisfied patients) caused by residual ametropia/astigmatism [98] or posterior capsular opacification (PCO), [97] although these subjective complains usually do not correspond to the objective VA [98, 142]. An additional cause of dissatisfaction is *dysphotopsia*, which is caused by the IOL itself or/and by a potential IOL decentration or IOL tilt or/and by a large pupil diameter. Refractive mIOLs appear to be related with higher levels of photic phenomena than diffractive mIOLs [143, 144]. Moreover, the existence of *dry eye disease* postoperatively found to be one of the patient complaints resulting in symptoms of discomfort, visual disturbance, and tear-film instability. Finally, *IOL explantation* has been reported in

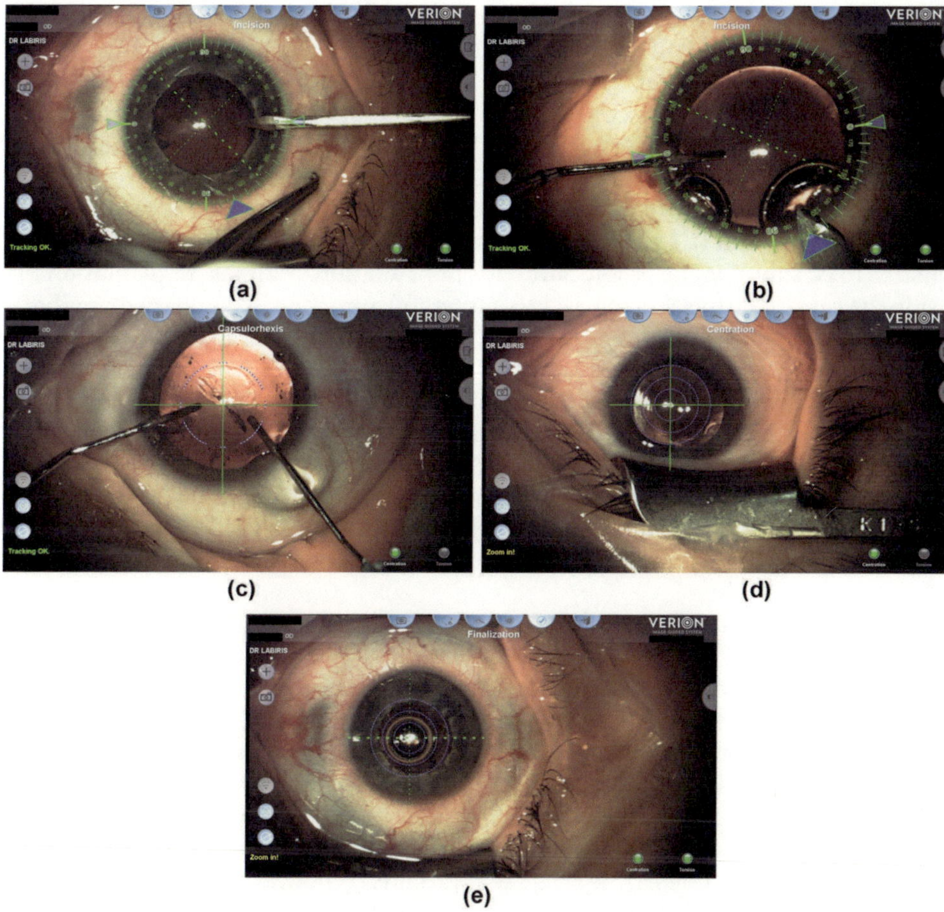

Figure 6.
The basic steps of multifocal IOL implantation using the Verion image-guided system ((a) sideport incisions, (b) main incision, (c) capsulorrhexis, (d) IOL centration, (e) finalization).

a frequency between 0.85% and 7 % [98, 145, 146] due to IOL dislocation, refractive error, PCO, failure to neuroadaptation [147] and, rarely, loss of normal color perception [148].

3.3 New IOL technologies for presbyopic correction

Apart from monovision technique with bilateral implantation of monofocal IOLs and bilateral implantation of multifocal IOLs, accommodative and EDOF IOL, as well as a combination of different IOL types and designs are some new alternative solutions of pseudophakic presbyopic correction. However, these options are beyond the scope of this chapter and they will not be analytically described.

3.3.1 Accommodative IOLs

Accommodative IOLs (aIOLs) are designed to simulate the mechanism of accommodation of the crystalline lens, which is capable of changing dynamically its dioptric power with accommodating effort, namely by modifying its shape after contraction of the ciliary muscle and providing functional vision at different distances [149].

AIOLs are still a developing field in the technology of premium IOLs where a variety of designs are still examined [150]. The mechanisms of action of the different types of aIOLs that are currently available are based on the three following principles: (a) change in axial position (i. single-optic aIOLs, and ii. dual-optic aIOLs), (b) change in shape or curvature, and (c) change in refractive index or power. Apart from the aforementioned aIOL designs, the following new design strategies of aIOLs, still in preclinical stage, have been proposed: (i) lens-filling aIOL techniques, and (ii) electroadaptive aIOLs [149, 151]. Another issue that remains to be solved is the best location for implantation of aIOLs. Implantation inside the capsular bag seem to be a less successful approach in comparison to the sulcus, since in sulcus, the dynamics from the ciliary body induce further movements of the IOL [149, 150].

Despite the significant development and evolution of aIOLs and the great variety of IOL designs, the majority of them are still in a development process and have shown some contradictory clinical data about their efficacy. The optimal aIOL with a broad range of accommodation still remains elusive, and different challenges exist for each lens design. However, new innovative and promising designs and technologies now exist having the restoration of accommodation as their common goal [149, 151].

3.3.2 Extended depth-of-focus (EDOF) IOLs

Extended depth-of-focus (EDOF) IOL is a new technology in the treatment of presbyopia-correcting IOLs. The basic optical principle of EDOF IOLs is to create a single elongated focal point, in contrast to monofocal IOLs, in which light is focused on one single point, and mIOLs, in which light is focused on two or three discrete points (**Figure 7**). In this way, EDOF IOLs eliminate the overlapping of far and near images caused my mIOLs, thus eliminating the halo effect. Specifically, EDOF IOLs provide a continuous focus range that extends from the far focus area until the intermediate distance, without the clearly asymmetric IOL power distribution that is provided by the mIOLs. In this way, EDOF IOLs avoid the presence of secondary out-of-focus images that originates the halos [152–154].

The idea of EDOF was first reported in 1984 by Nakazawa and Ohtsuki who measured an apparent 2.00 D accommodation in 39 pseudophakic eyes implanted with posterior chamber spherical IOLs and found a significant correlation between apparent accommodation and depth of field. This correlation was inversely proportional to the pupillary diameter [155]. After using multiple cornea- or IOL-based strategies, the first EDOF IOL (Symfony, Johnson and Johnson Vision, Jacksonville, FL) was introduced into the market receiving the European Economic Area

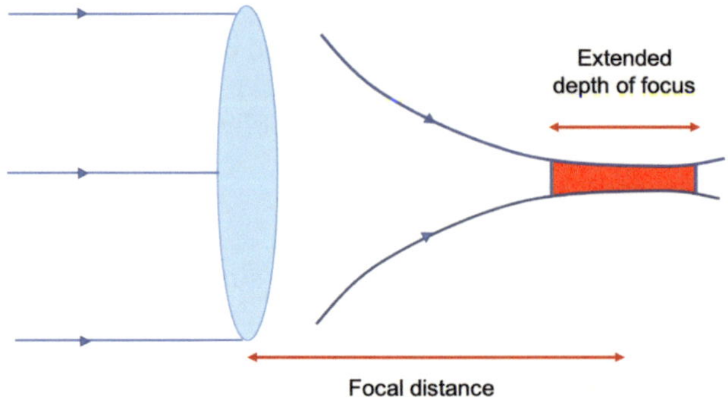

Figure 7.
EDOF IOL design.

certification mark in June 2014, and being approved by the United States Food and Drug Administration (FDA) in July 2016 [156].

Since then, a variety of EDOF-labeled IOLs have been released in the market and are based on the following 3 optical models: i) spherical aberration, ii) chromatic aberration, iii) pinhole effect, all of which allow obtaining greater depth of focus [157]. Apart from the pure EDOF IOLs, there are some IOLs that combine multifocality with low addition power and the EDOF technology, the so-called "hybrid IOLs" [157]. In general, EDOF IOLs provide better optical quality in comparison with monofocal and multifocal IOLs [158–160] Additionally, EDOF IOLs provide high uncorrected intermediate vision, but inadequate near vision [161, 162], thus allowing a relative spectacle independence. A potential disadvantage of EDOF-IOLs is a decreased quality of retinal image if the aberrations are excessively increased. Finally, contrast sensitivity, glare and halos vary depending on the EDOF-IOL technology, however, they seem to be better when compared to mIOLs. [163] Since the literature results about the optical performance of EDOF-IOLs are promising but contraindicating, [164–166] new large-scale studies need to be performed.

In any case, patients should be counseled about potential photic phenomena and the need for low power reading spectacles postoperatively. Moreover, the IOL type decision should be made depending on their profile and preferences.

3.3.3 Monovision techniques with combination of IOLs

When a large anisometropia is targeted for an optimal near visual acuity, pseudophakic monovision with implantation of monofocal IOLs results in a relative decrease in near stereopsis [49, 153]. Therefore, a new type of monovision with implantation of different IOL types and IOL technologies in each eye has been introduced. For instance, the implantation of a monofocal IOL in the dominant eye and a premium lens such as mIOL (bifocal or trifocal/refractive, diffractive or hybrid diffractive-refractive) [167, 168] or EDOF IOL in the recessive one, the so-called "hybrid monovision" or "mix and match" or "blended vision", has been applied and compared with the conventional myopic monovision techniques and with the binocular implantation of premium IOLs showing promising visual outcomes [153, 154, 169]. Additionally, the use of a refractive IOL in the dominant eye and a diffractive IOL in the recessive eye [170] or vice versa [171] has been reported showing very good visual outcomes including impressive spectacle independence at all distances and a contrast sensitivity being comparable with phakic patients. In general, it seems that hybrid monovision offers spectacle-free postoperative visual capacity at all distances with minimal optical phenomena.

4. Postoperative examination – follow-up

Apart from the full preoperative examination and the high-precision surgery that are necessary for optimal refractive outcomes in patients undergoing a pseudophakic presbyopic correction, especially with mIOLs, the postoperative follow-up plays an equally significant role in the best possible results. The most common follow-up timepoints are 1 day, 1 week, 1 month, 3 months, 6 months, 1 year, 2 years and so forth. Examination at the first postoperative day is commonly applied by many surgeons, However, the current literature supports that first-day examination after an uneventful phacoemulsification surgery is not necessary when patients have not posterior synechiae or chronic/recurrent uveitis and they are operated by experienced cataract surgeons. Thus, healthcare costs can be decreased without an increased risk to the patients [172].

A comprehensive postoperative examination should include primarily history, VA assessment, automatic (with auto-refractor) and manifest refraction, slit lamp biomicroscopy and IOP measurement. However, some additional examinations should be performed for the best possible evaluation of the visual performance and optical quality of vision, including defocus curves, contrast sensitivity assessment, corneal topography, aberrometry, pupillometry, and halometry or retinal straylight, if halos, glare and other photic phenomena are present [173]. Finally, patient satisfaction and potential photic phenomena should be assessed by history taking or, more specifically, through special quality of vision questionnaires [174–176]. Among them, some important aspects that should be taken into consideration are the following:

- *Visual acuity and refraction:* UDVA, BCDVA, UNVA, BCNVA, UIVA, and BCIVA should be included in the postoperative examination. Near and intermediate vision should be ideally evaluated with logarithmic printed or digital reading charts that evaluate not only reading acuity (RA), but also the maximum reading speed (MRS) and the critical print size (CPS), namely the smallest print size that can be read with the MRS [177–180]. *Defocus curves* could also be obtained. Apart from the manifest refraction, an auto-kerato-refractometer should be used.

- *Contrast sensitivity*: Contrast sensitivity under photopic and mesopic light conditions should ideally be assessed.

- *Slit lamp anterior segment examination:* Apart from the evaluation of the cornea (Seidel test, clarity), the anterior chamber (depth, inflammatory activity), and the pupil (shape, reactivity), in case of mIOL implantation, the centration of the mIOL should also be checked. Specifically, the coaxially sighted IOL light reflex (CSILR) should be identified by placing the slit illuminator in a coaxial position with the microscope, adjusting the narrow slit beam to a small rectangle and asking the patient to fixate on the slit lamp light. The light reflection on the mIOL indicates the position of the CSILR, which coincides with the visual axis, and ideally should fall on the central mIOL optic zone if the mIOL centration has been done according to the visual axis (**Figure 8**) [131].

- *Corneal topography and aberrometry:* Corneal topography and aberrometry are suggested to be performed postoperatively, since they might reveal potential residual astigmatism and aberrations, especially in case of postoperative dysphotopic phenomena at scotopic or mesopic light conditions.

- *Pupillometry:* Postoperative pupil diameter at photopic and mesopic light conditions and PCS are suggested to be measured, especially after implantation of mIOLs, in order potential dysphotopic phenomena to be explained and correlated with the objective pupil measurements.

As regards the surgery schedule of the fellow eye for a pseudophakic presbyopic correction, different factors described below should be taken into consideration:

- *Postoperative visual capacity (VA, reading speed, stereoscopic vision, dysphotopsia) and patient satisfaction:* After a successful lens extraction surgery, the surgeon should wait long enough for the patient's refraction to be stabilized and for the neuroadaptation process to take place, especially in case of dysphotopic phenomena. After this period of time, which can differ for each patient and each IOL design, [74] the surgeon could choose if and when the operation of

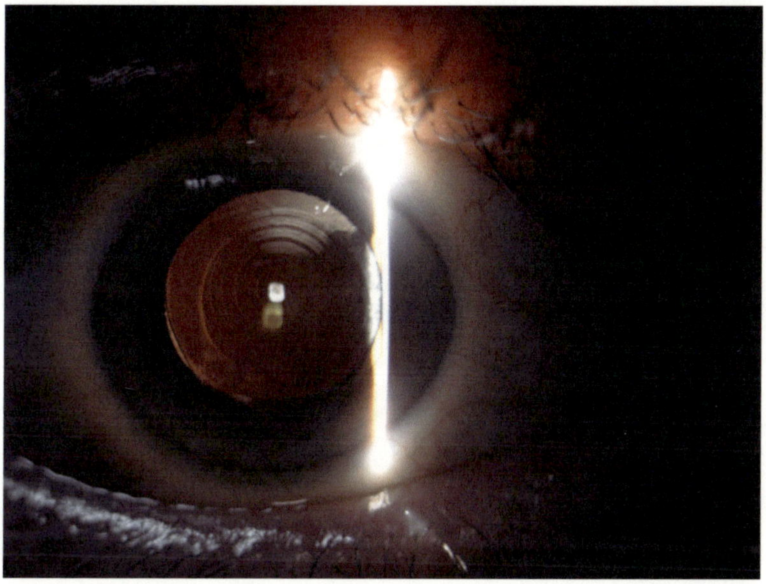

Figure 8.
Identification of the coaxially sighted IOL light reflex through slit lamp biomicroscopy following a multifocal IOL implantation.

the fellow eye could be performed, and the IOL design, as well. In addition, in case of patient dissatisfaction, the cause of dissatisfaction should be identified. If dysphotopsia or suboptimal near vision are the most serious patient's complaints, the surgeon should consider if the implantation of a different IOL design with fewer photic phenomena or with a near focus point could be the best option.

- *Patient's desire or not for lens extraction surgery at the fellow eye*

- *Crystalline lens clearance of the fellow eye:* In case of a clear crystalline lens, especially in young patients with unilateral cataract with a non-presbyopic fellow eye, the fellow eye may not require a lens extraction surgery for years or decades after the surgery of the first eye [181]. In fact, young people with a clear crystalline lens of the fellow eye seem to benefit from the avoidance of the fellow eye surgery, since the smooth transition among distant, intermediate and near vision that is provided by their clear non-presbyopic crystalline lens could not be equally replaced by an artificial IOL.

5. Conclusions

Pseudophakic presbyopic correction is now established as a safe and effective surgical method for the treatment of presbyopia, especially when it is combined with cataract. Pseudophakic presbyopic correction with monovision techniques, implantation of mIOL, aIOL or a combination of IOL designs is also related with excellent visual outcomes, improvement in vision and life quality, and high patient satisfaction. Rapid technological advances have led to an increase in the number of the available IOL technologies and presbyopia correction techniques. Additionally, advances and innovation in imaging and preoperative assessment, but also the high precision that is provided pre- and intraoperatively by image-guided systems, have allowed customized selection of IOLs and presbyopia correction strategies according to visual demands and activities, personality and special anatomical eye characteristics. Finally, since the research on IOL technologies is constantly evolving, the introduction of new promising IOL designs and the improvement of the already existing IOLs are expected within the next decade.

Conflict of interest

The authors declare no conflict of interest.

Author details

Georgios Labiris* and Eirini-Kanella Panagiotopoulou
Department of Ophthalmology, University Hospital of Alexandroupolis, Alexandroupolis, Greece

*Address all correspondence to: labiris@usa.net

References

[1] Lu Q, Congdon N, He X, Murthy GVS, Yang A, He W. Quality of life and near vision impairment due to functional presbyopia among rural Chinese adults. Invest Ophthalmol Vis Sci. 2011;52(7):4118-4123. DOI: 10.1167/iovs.10-6353

[2] Alió JL, Plaza-Puche AB, Piñero DP, Amparo F, Jiménez R, Rodríguez-Prats JL, Javaloy J, Pongo V. Optical analysis, reading performance, and quality-of-life evaluation after implantation of a diffractive multifocal intraocular lens. J Cataract Refract Surg. 2011;37(1):27-37. DOI: 10.1016/j.jcrs.2010.07.035

[3] Frick KD, Joy SM, Wilson DA, Naidoo KS, Holden BA. The global burden of potential productivity loss from uncorrected presbyopia. Ophthalmology. 2015;122(8):1706-1710. DOI: 10.1016/j.ophtha.2015.04.014

[4] Chou KL. Combined effect of vision and hearing impairment on depression in older adults: evidence from the English Longitudinal Study of Ageing. J Affect Disord. 2008;106(1-2):191-196. DOI: 10.1016/j.jad.2007.05.028

[5] Luo BP, Brown GC, Luo SC, Brown MM. The quality of life associated with presbyopia. Am J Ophthalmol. 2008;145(4):618-622. DOI: 10.1016/j.ajo.2007.12.011

[6] Sharma B, Abell RG, Arora T, Antony T, Vajpayee RB. Techniques of anterior capsulotomy in cataract surgery. Indian J Ophthalmol. 2019;67(4):450-460. DOI: 10.4103/ijo.IJO_1728_18

[7] Gil-Cazorla R, Shah S, Naroo SA. A review of the surgical options for the correction of presbyopia. Br J Ophthalmol. 2016;100(1):62-70. DOI: 10.1136/bjophthalmol-2015-306663

[8] Mahrous A, Ciralsky JP, Lai EC. Revisiting monovision for presbyopia. Curr Opin Ophthalmol. 2018; 29(4):313-317. DOI:10.1097/icu.0000000000000487

[9] Labiris G, Ntonti P, Patsiamanidi M, Sideroudi H, Georgantzoglou K, Kozobolis VP. Evaluation of activities of daily living following pseudophakic presbyopic correction. Eye Vis (Lond). 2017;4:2. DOI: 10.1186/s40662-016-0067-1

[10] Xiao J, Jiang C, Zhang M. Pseudophakic monovision is an important surgical approach to being spectacle-free. Indian J Ophthalmol. 2011;59(6):481-485. DOI: 10.4103/0301-4738.86318

[11] Zhang F, Sugar A, Jacobsen G, Collins M. Visual function and spectacle independence after cataract surgery: bilateral diffractive multifocal intraocular lenses versus monovision pseudophakia. J Cataract Refract Surg. 2011;37(5):853-858. DOI: 10.1016/j.jcrs.2010.12.041

[12] Zettl S, Reiß S, Terwee T, Guthoff RF, Beck R, Stachs O. Der Effekt der pseudophaken Minimonovision als Option einer Brillenunabhängigkeit im Alltag [Effect of pseudophacic mini-monovision as an option for independence of spectacles in everyday life]. Klin Monbl Augenheilkd. 2014;231(12):1196-1202. German. DOI: 10.1055/s-0034-1383367

[13] Braga-Mele R, Chang D, Dewey S, Foster G, Henderson BA, Hill W, Hoffman R, Little B, Mamalis N, Oetting T, Serafano D, Talley-Rostov A, Vasavada A, Yoo S; ASCRS Cataract Clinical Committee. Multifocal intraocular lenses: relative indications and contraindications for implantation. J Cataract Refract Surg. 2014;40(2):313-322. DOI: 10.1016/j.jcrs.2013.12.011

[14] Liu YC, Wilkins M, Kim T, Malyugin B, Mehta JS. Cataracts. Lancet. 2017;390(10094):600-612. DOI: 10.1016/S0140-6736(17)30544-5

[15] Malyugin B. Cataract surgery in small pupils. Indian J Ophthalmol. 2017;65(12):1323-1328. DOI: 10.4103/ijo.IJO_800_17

[16] Lin HY, Chen HY, Fam HB, Chuang YJ, Yeoh R, Lin PJ. Comparison of corneal power obtained from VERION image-guided surgery system and four other devices. Clin Ophthalmol. 2017;11:1291-1299. DOI: 10.2147/OPTH.S137878

[17] Srivannaboon S, Chirapapaisan C. Comparison of refractive outcomes using conventional keratometry or total keratometry for IOL power calculation in cataract surgery. Graefes Arch Clin Exp Ophthalmol. 2019;257(12):2677-2682. DOI: 10.1007/s00417-019-04443-7

[18] Lawless M, Jiang JY, Hodge C, Sutton G, Roberts TV, Barrett G. Total keratometry in intraocular lens power calculations in eyes with previous laser refractive surgery. Clin Exp Ophthalmol. 2020;48(6):749-756. DOI: 10.1111/ceo.13760

[19] Fabian E, Wehner W. Prediction Accuracy of Total Keratometry Compared to Standard Keratometry Using Different Intraocular Lens Power Formulas. J Refract Surg. 2019;35(6):362-368. DOI: 10.3928/1081597X-20190422-02

[20] Jack T. Holladay, IOL Power Calculations for Multifocal Lenses. Cataract & Refractive Surgery Today, 2007. Available from: https://crstoday.com/articles/2007-aug/crst0807_11-php/ [Accessed: 2021-01-06]

[21] Kelly SP, Jalil A. Wrong intraocular lens implant; learning from reported patient safety incidents. Eye (Lond). 2011;25(6):730-734. DOI: 10.1038/eye.2011.22

[22] Kansal V, Schlenker M, Ahmed IIK. Interocular Axial Length and Corneal Power Differences as Predictors of Postoperative Refractive Outcomes after Cataract Surgery. Ophthalmology. 2018;125(7):972-981. DOI: 10.1016/j.ophtha.2018.01.021

[23] Findl O, Kriechbaum K, Sacu S, Kiss B, Polak K, Nepp J, Schild G, Rainer G, Maca S, Petternel V, Lackner B, Drexler W. Influence of operator experience on the performance of ultrasound biometry compared to optical biometry before cataract surgery. J Cataract Refract Surg. 2003;29:1950-1955. DOI: 10.1016/s0886-3350(03)00243-8

[24] Li Y, Li HX, Liu YC, et al. Comparison of immersion ultrasound and low coherence reflectometry for ocular biometry in cataract patients. Int J Ophthalmol. 2018;11(6):966-969. DOI:10.18240/ijo.2018.06.11

[25] Ademola-Popoola DS, Nzeh DA, Saka SE, Olokoba LB, Obajolowo TS. Comparison of ocular biometry measurements by applanation and immersion A-scan techniques. J Curr Ophthalmol. 2016;27(3-4):110-114. DOI:10.1016/j.joco.2015.12.002

[26] Ventura AC, Wälti R, Böhnke M. Corneal thickness and endothelial density before and after cataract surgery. Br J Ophthalmol. 2001;85(1):18-20. DOI: 10.1136/bjo.85.1.18

[27] Beiko GHH. The Fundamentals of Spherical Aberration. Cataract & Refractive Surgery Today (Europe). 2012. Available from: https://crstodayeurope.com/articles/2012-jul/the-fundamentals-of-spherical-aberration/ [Accessed: 2021-01-21]

[28] Wang L, Dai E, Koch DD, Nathoo A. Optical aberrations of the

human anterior cornea. J Cataract Refract Surg. 2003;29(8):1514-1521. DOI: 10.1016/s0886-3350(03)00467-x

[29] Visser N, Berendschot TT, Verbakel F, Tan AN, de Brabander J, Nuijts RM. Evaluation of the comparability and repeatability of four wavefront aberrometers. Invest Ophthalmol Vis Sci. 2011;52(3):1302-1311. DOI: 10.1167/iovs.10-5841

[30] Atchison DA, Suheimat M, Mathur A, Lister LJ, Rozema J. Anterior Corneal, Posterior Corneal, and Lenticular Contributions to Ocular Aberrations. Invest Ophthalmol Vis Sci. 2016 Oct 1;57(13):5263-5270. DOI: 10.1167/iovs.16-20067

[31] Fu Y, Kou J, Chen D, Wang D, Zhao Y, Hu M, Lin X, Dai Q, Li J, Zhao YE. Influence of angle kappa and angle alpha on visual quality after implantation of multifocal intraocular lenses. J Cataract Refract Surg. 2019;45(9):1258-1264. DOI: 10.1016/j.jcrs.2019.04.003

[32] Mabed IS, Saad A, Guilbert E, Gatinel D. Measurement of pupil center shift in refractive surgery candidates with caucasian eyes using infrared pupillometry. J Refract Surg. 2014;30(10):694-700. DOI: 10.3928/1081597X-20140903-07

[33] Tchah H, Nam K, Yoo A. Predictive factors for photic phenomena after refractive, rotationally asymmetric, multifocal intraocular lens implantation. Int J Ophthalmol. 2017;10(2):241-245. DOI:10.18240/ijo.2017.02.10

[34] Fischinger I, Seiler TG, Schmidinger G, Seiler T. Verschiebung des Pupillenzentroids : Marketing oder klinisch relevanter Parameter? [Pupil centroid shift: Marketing tool or essential clinical parameter?]. Ophthalmologe. 2015;112(8):661-4. German. DOI: 10.1007/s00347-014-3170-5

[35] Duman R, Tok Çevik M, Görkem Çevik S, Duman R, Perente İ. Corneal endothelial cell density in healthy Caucasian population. Saudi J Ophthalmol. 2016;30(4):236-239. DOI: 10.1016/j.sjopt.2016.10.003

[36] Bamdad S, Bolkheir A, Sedaghat MR, Motamed M. Changes in corneal thickness and corneal endothelial cell density after phacoemulsification cataract surgery: a double-blind randomized trial. Electron Physician. 2018;10(4):6616-6623. DOI: 10.19082/6616

[37] Mishima S. Clinical investigations on the corneal endothelium-XXXVIII Edward Jackson Memorial Lecture. Am J Ophthalmol. 1982;93(1):1-29. DOI: 10.1016/0002-9394(82)90693-6

[38] Edelhauser HF. The balance between corneal transparency and edema: the Proctor Lecture. Invest Ophthalmol Vis Sci. 2006;47(5):1754-1767. DOI: 10.1167/iovs.05-1139

[39] Yoo YS, Whang WJ, Kim HS, Joo CK, Yoon G. Preoperative biometric measurements with anterior segment optical coherence tomography and prediction of postoperative intraocular lens position. Medicine (Baltimore). 2019;98(50):e18026. DOI: 10.1097/MD.0000000000018026

[40] Goto S, Maeda N, Koh S, Ohnuma K, Hayashi K, Iehisa I, Noda T, Nishida K. Prediction of Postoperative Intraocular Lens Position with Angle-to-Angle Depth Using Anterior Segment Optical Coherence Tomography. Ophthalmology. 2016;123(12):2474-2480. DOI: 10.1016/j.ophtha.2016.09.005

[41] Panagiotopoulou EK, Ntonti P, Gkika M, Konstantinidis A, Perente I, Dardabounis D, Ioannakis K, Labiris G. Image-guided lens extraction surgery: a systematic review. Int J Ophthalmol. 2019;12(1):135-151. DOI: 10.18240/ijo.2019.01.21

[42] Boerner CF, Thrasher BH. Results of monovision correction in bilateral pseudophakes. J Am Intraocul Implant Soc. 1984; 10:49-50. DOI: 10.1016/s0146-2776(84)80077-4

[43] Zhang F. Potential Concerns and Contraindications for IOL Monovision. Clin Surg. 2016;1:1084.

[44] Zhang F. Pseudophakic Monovision (A Clinical Guide). 1st ed. New York, Stuttgart, Delhi, Rio de Janeiro: Thieme; 2018.

[45] European Society of Cataract and Refractive Surgery Clinical Survey Results, 2016. Available from: http://www.eurotimes.org/escrs-clinical-survey-2016-results/ [Accessed: 2021-12-14]

[46] Goldberg DG, Goldberg MH, Shah R, Meagher JN, Ailani H. Pseudophakic mini-monovision: high patient satisfaction, reduced spectacle dependence, and low cost. BMC Ophthalmology 2018;18(1):293. DOI: 10.1186/s12886-018-0963-3

[47] Labiris G, Giarmoukakis A, Patsiamanidi M, Papadopoulos Z, Kozobolis VP. Mini-monovision versus multifocal intraocular lens implantation. J Cataract Refract Surg 2015;41(1):53-57.

[48] Labiris G, Toli A, Perente A, Ntonti P, Kozobolis VP. A systematic review of pseudophakic monovision for presbyopia correction. Int J Ophthalmol 2017;10(6):992-1000. DOI: 10.1016/j.jcrs.2014.06.015

[49] Ito M, Shimizu K. Pseudophakic monovision. Careful patient selection is crucial. Cataract & Refractive Surgery Today (Europe) 2009;(Oct):64-66. Available from: https://crstodayeurope.com/articles/2009-oct/1009_14-php/ [Accessed: 2021-01-21]

[50] Handa T, Mukuno K, Uozato H, Niida T, Shoji N, Minei R, Nitta M, Shimizu K. Ocular dominance and patient satisfaction after monovision induced by intraocular lens implantation. J Cataract Refract Surg. 2004;30(4):769-774. DOI: 10.1016/j.jcrs.2003.07.013

[51] American Academy of Ophthalmology, Monovision should be induced cautiously in patients with strabismus history. 2011. Available from: https://www.aao.org/editors-choice/monovision-should-be-induced-cautiously-in-patient [Accessed: 2021-01-17]

[52] Ito M, Shimizu K, Amano R, Handa T. Assessment of visual performance in pseudophakic monovision. J Cataract Refract Surg. 2009;35(4):710-714. DOI: 10.1016/j.jcrs.2008.12.019

[53] Finkelman YM, Ng JQ, Barrett GD. Patient satisfaction and visual function after pseudophakic monovision. J Cataract Refract Surg. 2009;35(6):998-1002.

[54] Burge J, Rodriguez-Lopez V, Dorronsoro C. Monovision and the Misperception of Motion. Curr Biol. 2019;29(15):2586-2592.e4. DOI:10.1016/j.cub.2019.06.070

[55] Smith CE, Allison RS, Wilkinson F, Wilcox LM. Monovision: Consequences for depth perception from large disparities. Exp Eye Res. 2019;183:62-67. DOI: 10.1016/j.exer.2018.09.005

[56] Hoffer KJ. Personal history in bifocal intraocular lenses, (Chapter 12). In: Maxwell A, Nordan LT, eds. Current Concepts of Multifocal Intraocular Lenses. Thorofare: Slack, Inc; 1991:127e132.

[57] Pearce JL. Multifocal intraocular lenses. Curr Opin Ophthalmol. 1997;8(1):2-5.

[58] Zvorničanin J, Zvorničanin E. Premium intraocular lenses: The past,

present and future. J Curr Ophthalmol. 2018;30(4):287-296. DOI: 10.1016/j.joco.2018.04.003

[59] Davison JA, Simpson MJ. History and development of the apodized diffractive intraocular lens. J Cataract Refract Surg. 2006;32:849-858 DOI: 10.1016/j.jcrs.2006.02.006

[60] Schwiegerling J, Petznick A. Refractive and Diffractive Principles in Presbyopia-Correcting IOLs — An Optical Lesson. Alcon. Available from: https://us.alconscience.com/wp-content/uploads/2020/10/Refractive-and-Diffractive-Principles-in-Presbyopia-Correcting-IOLs-An-Optical-Lesson-US-REF-1900001.pdf [Accessed: 2021-01-17]

[61] Rampat R, Gatinel D. Multifocal and Extended Depth-of-Focus Intraocular Lenses in 2020. Ophthalmology. 2020:S0161-6420(20)30931-3. DOI: 10.1016/j.ophtha.2020.09.026

[62] Gooi P, Ahmed IK. Review of presbyopic IOLs: multifocal and accommodating IOLs. Int Ophthalmol Clin. 2012 Spring;52(2):41-50. DOI: 10.1097/IIO.0b013e31824b87be

[63] Moreno V, Román JF, Salgueiro JR. High efficiency diffractive lenses: Deduction of kinoform profile. American Journal of Physics 1997;65:556-562. DOI: 10.1119/1.18587

[64] Alió JL, Pikkel J. Multifocal Intraocular Lenses. The Art and the Practice. 2nd ed. Switzerland: Springer Nature; 2019. DOI: 10.1007/978-3-030-21282-7

[65] Acrysof IQ Restor, Model SN6AD1 – Product Information. Available from: https://www.alcon.com/eye-care-products [Accessed: 2021-02-08]

[66] Acrysof IQ Restor, Product information, Alcon Laboratories, Inc. Available from: https://www.accessdata.fda.gov/cdrh_docs/pdf4/P040020S050d.pdf. [Accessed: 2021-02-08]

[67] Intraocular lenses, PhysIOL. Available from: https://www.physiol.eu/en-US/Products/Intraocular-lenses [Accessed: 2021-02-08]

[68] Kim MJ, Zheleznyak L, Macrae S, Tchah H, Yoon G. Objective evaluation of through-focus optical performance of presbyopia-correcting intraocular lenses using an optical bench system. J Cataract Refract Surg. 2011;37(7):1305-1312. DOI: 10.1016/j.jcrs.2011.03.033

[69] AcrySof IQ PanOptix, Summary of Safety and Effectiveness data. Fort Worth, TX: Alcon Laboratories, Inc. 2019. Available from: https://www.accessdata.fda.gov/cdrh_docs/pdf4/P040020S087B.pdf [Accessed: 2021-02-08]

[70] Intraocular lenses. Precision Lens. Available from: https://www.precisionlens.net/products/jj-vision-products/lenses/ [Accessed: 2021-02-08]

[71] Zeiss AT LISA 809M. Technical Specifications. Available from: https://www.zeiss.com/meditec/int/product-portfolio/iols/multifocal-iols/at-lisa-809m.html [Accessed: 2021-02-08]

[72] Zeiss AT LISA tri 839MP preloaded. Technical Specifications. Available from: https://www.zeiss.com/meditec/int/product-portfolio/iols/multifocal-iols/at-lisa-tri-family.html [Accessed: 2021-02-08]

[73] Rudalevicius P, Lekaviciene R, Auffarth GU, Liutkeviciene R, Jasinskas V. Relations between patient personality and patients' dissatisfaction after multifocal intraocular lens implantation: clinical study based on the five factor inventory personality evaluation. Eye (Lond). 2020;34(4):717-724. DOI: 10.1038/s41433-019-0585-x

[74] Mester U, Vaterrodt T, Goes F, Huetz W, Neuhann I, Schmickler S, Szurman P, Gekeler K. Impact of personality characteristics on patient satisfaction after multifocal intraocular lens implantation: results from the "happy patient study". J Refract Surg. 2014;30(10):674-678. DOI: 10.3928/1081597X-20140903-05

[75] Al-Shymali O, Alió JL. Neuroadaptation Failure Corrected by Exchanging with a Different Multifocal Intraocular Lens. In: Alió JL, Pikkel J, editors. Multifocal Intraocular Lenses. The Art and the Practice. 2nd ed. Switzerland: Springer Nature; 2019. p. 111-119. DOI: 10.1007/978-3-030-21282-7_11

[76] Kelly SP, Jalil A. Wrong intraocular lens implant; learning from reported patient safety incidents. Eye (Lond). 2011;25(6):730-734. DOI: 10.1038/eye.2011.22

[77] Holladay JT, Prager TC, Chandler TY, Musgrove KH, Lewis JW, Ruiz RS. A three part system for refining intraocular lens power calculations. J Cataract Refract Surg. 1988;13:17-24. DOI: 10.1016/s0886-3350(88)80059-2

[78] Retzalff JA, Sanders DR, Kraff MC. Development of the SRK/T intraocular lens implant power calculation formula. J Cataract Refract Surg. 1990;16:333-340. DOI: 10.1016/s0886-3350(13)80705-5

[79] Hoffer KJ. The Hoffer Q formula: a comparison of theoretic and regression formulas. J Cataract Refract Surg. 1993;19:700-712. DOI: 10.1016/s0886-3350(13)80338-0

[80] Eom Y, Kang SY, Song JS, Kim YY, Kim HM, Comparison of Hoffer Q and Haigis formulae for intraocular lens power calculation according to the anterior chamber depth in short eyes. Am J Ophthalmol. 2014;157(4):818-824.e2. DOI: 10.1016/j.ajo.2013.12.017

[81] Moschos MM, Chatziralli IP, Koutsandrea C. Intraocular lens power calculation in eyes with short axial length. Indian J Ophthalmol. 2014;62(6):692-694. DOI:10.4103/0301-4738.129791

[82] Savini G, Taroni L, Hoffer KJ. Recent developments in intraocular lens power calculation methods-update 2020. Ann Transl Med. 2020;8(22):1553. DOI:10.21037/atm-20-2290

[83] Petermeier K, Gekeler F, Messias A, Spitzer MS, Haigis W, Szurman P. Intraocular lens power calculation and optimized constants for highly myopic eyes. J Cataract Refract Surg. 2009; 35(9):1575-8151. DOI: 10.1016/j.jcrs.2009.04.028

[84] Kane JX, Van Heerden A, Atik A, Petsoglou C. Intraocular lens power formula accuracy: Comparison of 7 formulas. J Cataract Refract Surg. 2016;42(10):1490-1500. DOI: 10.1016/j.jcrs.2016.07.021

[85] Liu J, Wang L, Chai F, Han Y, Qian S, Koch DD, Weikert MP. Comparison of intraocular lens power calculation formulas in Chinese eyes with axial myopia. J Cataract Refract Surg. 2019;45(6):725-731. DOI: 10.1016/j.jcrs.2019.01.018

[86] Dong J, Zhang Y, Zhang H, Jia Z, Zhang S, Wang X. Comparison of axial length, anterior chamber depth and intraocular lens power between IOLMaster and ultrasound in normal, long and short eyes. PloS One. 2018;13(3):e0194273. DOI: 10.1371/journal.pone.0194273

[87] Cech R, Utíkal T, Juhászová J. Srovnání optické a ultrazvukové biometrie a zhodnocení užívání obou metod v praxi [Comparison of optical and ultrasound biometry and assessment of using both methods in practice]. Cesk Slov Oftalmol. 2014;70(1):3-9. Czech.

[88] Kolega MŠ, Kovačević S, Čanović S, Pavičić AD, Bašić JK. Comparison of IOL—master and ultrasound biometry in preoperative intra ocular lens (IOL) power calculation. Coll Antropol. 2015;39(1):233-235.

[89] Kieval JZ, Al-Hashimi S, Davidson RS, Hamilton DR, Jackson MA, LaBorwit S, Patterson LE, Stonecipher KG, Donaldson K; ASCRS Refractive Cataract Surgery Subcommittee. Prevention and management of refractive prediction errors following cataract surgery. J Cataract Refract Surg. 2020;46(8):1189-1197. DOI: 10.1097/j.jcrs.0000000000000269

[90] Carones F. Residual astigmatism threshold and patient satisfaction with bifocal, trifocal, and extended range of vision intraocular lenses (IOLs). Open J Ophthalmol. 2017;7(1):1-7. DOI: 10.4236/ojoph.2017.71001

[91] Eyeworld Supplements. The American Society of Cataract and Refractive Surgery Clinical Survey. 2018. Available from: https://supplements.eyeworld.org/eyeworld-supplements/december-2018-clinical-survey [Accessed: 2021-01-21]

[92] Kaur M, Shaikh F, Falera R, Titiyal JS. Optimizing outcomes with toric intraocular lenses. Indian J Ophthalmol. 2017;65(12):1301-1313. DOI:10.4103/ijo.IJO_810_17

[93] Bryan SL. IOL Power Calculations for Eyes With Astigmatism. Advanced Clinical Cases. Available from: https://collaborativeeye.com/articles/advanced-clinical-cases-2/iol-power-calculations-for-eyes-with-astigmatism/ [Accessed: 2021-01-17]

[94] Abulafia A, Barrett GD, Kleinmann G, et al. Prediction of refractive outcomes with toric intraocular lens implantation. J Cataract Refract Surg. 2015;41(5):936-944. DOI: 10.1016/j.jcrs.2014.08.036

[95] Salati C, Salvetat ML, Zeppieri M, Brusini P. Pupil size influence on the intraocular performance of the multifocal AMO-Array intraocular lens in elderly patients. Eur J Ophthalmol. 2007;17(4):571-578. DOI: 10.1177/112067210701700415

[96] Park CY, Oh SY, Chuck RS. Measurement of angle kappa and centration in refractive surgery. Curr Opin Ophthalmol. 2012;23(4):269-275. DOI: 10.1097/ICU.0b013e3283543c41

[97] Woodward MA, Randleman JB, Stulting RD. Dissatisfaction after multifocal intraocular lens implantation. J Cataract Refract Surg. 2009;35(6):992-997. DOI: 10.1016/j.jcrs.2009.01.031

[98] de Vries NE, Webers CA, Touwslager WR, Bauer NJ, de Brabander J, Berendschot TT, Nuijts RM. Dissatisfaction after implantation of multifocal intraocular lenses. J Cataract Refract Surg. 2011;37(5):859-865. DOI: 10.1016/j.jcrs.2010.11.032

[99] Pepin SM. Neuroadaptation of presbyopia-correcting intraocular lenses. Curr Opin Ophthalmol. 2008;19(1):10-12. DOI: 10.1097/ICU.0b013e3282f31758

[100] Tchah H, Nam K, Yoo A. Predictive factors for photic phenomena after refractive, rotationally asymmetric, multifocal intraocular lens implantation. Int J Ophthalmol. 2017;10(2):241-245. DOI:10.18240/ijo.2017.02.10

[101] Rosales P, De Castro A, Jiménez-alfaro I, Marcos S. Intraocular lens alignment from purkinje and Scheimpflug imaging. Clin Exp Optom, 2010;93:400-408. DOI: 10.1111/j.1444-0938.2010.00514.x

[102] Prakash G, Prakash DR, Agarwal A, Kumar DA, Agarwal A, Jacob S. Predictive factor and kappa angle analysis for visual satisfactions

in patients with multifocal IOL implantation. Eye (Lond). 2011;25:1187-1193. DOI: 10.1038/eye.2011.150

[103] Fu Y, Kou J, Chen D, Wang D, Zhao Y, Hu M, Lin X, Dai Q, Li J, Zhao YE. Influence of angle kappa and angle alpha on visual quality after implantation of multifocal intraocular lenses. J Cataract Refract Surg. 2019;45(9):1258-1264. DOI: 10.1016/j.jcrs.2019.04.003

[104] Moshirfar M, Hoggan RN, Muthappan V. Angle Kappa and its importance in refractive surgery. Oman J Ophthalmol, 2013;6:151-158. DOI: 10.4103/0974-620X.122268

[105] Soda M, Yaguchi S. Effect of decentration on the optical performance in multifocal intraocular lenses. Ophthalmologica. 2012;227(4):197-204. DOI: 10.1159/000333820

[106] Asim R. Piracha. Using angle alpha in premium IOL screening. A simple measurement can give you a better sense of how well the IOL will center over the visual axis postoperatively. Available from: https://crstoday.com/wp-content/themes/crst/assets/downloads/crst0316_cs_Piracha.pdf. [Accessed: 2021-02-08]

[107] Visser N, Nuijts RMMA, de Vries NE, Bauer NJV. Visual outcomes and patient satisfaction after cataract surgery with toric multifocal intraocular lens implantation. J Cataract Refract Surg. 2011; 37:2034-2042. DOI: 10.1159/000333820

[108] Hamza I, Aly MG, Hashem KA. Multifocal IOL dissatisfaction in patients with high coma aberrations. Presented at: ASCRS Symposium on Cataract, IOL and Refractive Surgery; 27 March 2011; San Diego, California, USA.

[109] Velasco-Barona C, Corredor-Ortega C, Mendez-Leon A, Casillas-Chavarín NL, Valdepeña-López Velarde D, Cervantes-Coste G, Malacara-Hernández D, Gonzalez-Salinas R. Influence of Angle κ and Higher-Order Aberrations on Visual Quality Employing Two Diffractive Trifocal IOLs. J Ophthalmol. 2019;2019:7018937. DOI: 10.1155/2019/7018937

[110] Atchison DA, Mathur A. Effects of pupil center shift on ocular aberrations. Invest Ophthalmol Vis Sci. 2014;55(9):5862-5870. DOI: 10.1167/iovs.14-14212

[111] Liao X, Lin J, Tian J, Wen B, Tan Q, Lan C. Evaluation of Optical Quality: Ocular Scattering and Aberrations in Eyes Implanted with Diffractive Multifocal or Monofocal Intraocular Lenses. Curr Eye Res. 2018;43(6):696-701. DOI: 10.1080/02713683.2018.1449220

[112] Donnenfeld ED, Solomon R, Roberts CW, Wittpenn JR, McDonald MB, Perry HD. Cyclosporine 0.05% to improve visual outcomes after multifocal intraocular lens implantation. J Cataract Refract Surg. 2010;36:1095-1100. DOI: 10.1016/j.jcrs.2009.12.049

[113] Garg P, Gupta A, Tandon N, Raj P. Dry Eye Disease after Cataract Surgery: Study of its Determinants and Risk Factors. Turk J Ophthalmol. 2020;50(3):133-142. DOI:10.4274/tjo.galenos.2019.45538

[114] Li XM, Hu L, Hu J, Wang W. Investigation of dry eye disease and analysis of the pathogenic factors in patients after cataract surgery. Cornea. 2007;26:S16–S20. DOI: 10.1097/ICO.0b013e31812f67ca

[115] Alio JL, Colecha JR, Pastor S, Rodriguez A, Artola A. Symptomatic dry eye treatment with autologous platelet-rich plasma. Ophthalmic Res. 2007;39:124-129. DOI: 10.1159/000100933

[116] Alio JL, Arnalich-Montiel F, Rodriguez AE. The role of "eye platelet rich plasma" (E-PRP) for wound healing in ophthalmology. Curr Pharm Biotechnol. 2012;13:1257-1265. DOI: 10.2174/138920112800624355

[117] Pepose JS. Maximizing satisfaction with presbyopia correcting intraocular lenses: the missing link. Am J Ophthalmol. 2008;146:641-648. DOI: 10.1016/j.ajo.2008.07.033

[118] Makhotkina NY, Nijkamp MD, Berendschot TTJM, van den Borne B, Nuijts RMMA. Effect of active evaluation on the detection of negative dysphotopsia after sequential cataract surgery: discrepancy between incidences of unsolicited and solicited complaints. Acta Ophthalmol. 2018;96(1):81-87. DOI: 10.1111/aos.13508

[119] Khor WB, Afshari NA. The role of presbyopia-correcting intraocular lenses after laser in situ keratomileusis. Curr Opin Ophthalmol. 2013;24(1):35-40. DOI: 10.1097/ICU.0b013e32835ab457

[120] Vrijman V, Abulafia A, van der Linden JW, van der Meulen IJE, Mourits MP, Lapid-Gortzak R. ASCRS calculator formula accuracy in multifocal intraocular lens implantation in hyperopic corneal refractive laser surgery eyes. J Cataract Refract Surg. 2019;45(5):582-586. DOI: 10.1016/j.jcrs.2018.12.006

[121] Vrijman V, van der Linden JW, van der Meulen IJE, Mourits MP, Lapid-Gortzak R. Multifocal intraocular lens implantation after previous hyperopic corneal refractive laser surgery. J Cataract Refract Surg. 2018;44(4):466-470. DOI: 10.1016/j.jcrs.2018.01.030

[122] Hoffer KJ. Intraocular lens power calculation for eyes after refractive keratotomy. J Refract Surg. 1995;11(6):490-493.

[123] Holladay JT. Consultations in refractive surgery. Refract Corneal Surg. 1989; 5:203

[124] Wang L, Hill WE, Koch DD. Evaluation of intraocular lens power prediction methods using the American Society of Cataract and Refractive Surgeons post-keratorefractive intraocular lens power calculator. J Cataract Refract Surg 2010; 36:1466-1473. DOI: 10.1016/j.jcrs.2010.03.044

[125] Vrijman V, Abulafia A, van der Linden JW, van der Meulen IJE, Mourits MP, Lapid-Gortzak R. Evaluation of Different IOL Calculation Formulas of the ASCRS Calculator in Eyes After Corneal Refractive Laser Surgery for Myopia With Multifocal IOL Implantation. J Refract Surg. 2019;35(1):54-59. DOI: 10.3928/1081597X-20181119-01

[126] Vrijman V, Abulafia A, van der Linden JW, van der Meulen IJE, Mourits MP, Lapid-Gortzak R. ASCRS calculator formula accuracy in multifocal intraocular lens implantation in hyperopic corneal refractive laser surgery eyes. J Cataract Refract Surg. 2019;45(5):582-586. DOI: 10.1016/j.jcrs.2018.12.006

[127] Panagiotopoulou EK, Ntonti P, Vlachou E, Georgantzoglou K, Labiris G. Patients' Expectations in Lens Extraction Surgery: a Systematic Review. Acta Medica (Hradec Kralove). 2018;61(4):115-124. DOI: 10.14712/18059694.2018.129

[128] Baek T, Lee K, Kagaya F, Tomidokoro A, Amano S, Oshika T. Factors affecting the forward shift of posterior corneal surface after laser in situ keratomileusis. Ophthalmology. 2001 Feb;108(2):317-320. DOI: 10.1016/s0161-6420(00)00502-9

[129] Christopher Kent. Choosing the Best IOL For a Nonstandard Eye. Review of Ophthalmology. 2016. Available from:

https://www.reviewofophthalmology.com/article/choosing-the-best-iol-for-a-nonstandard-eye [Accessed: 2021-01-20]

[130] Alió JL, Pikkel J. Multifocal Intraocular Lenses and Corneal Refractive Surgery. In: Alió JL, Pikkel J, editors. Multifocal Intraocular Lenses. The Art and the Practice. 2nd ed. Switzerland: Springer Nature; 2019. p. 67-72. DOI: 10.1007/978-3-030-21282-7_11

[131] Melki SA, Harissi-Dagher M. Coaxially sighted intraocular lens light reflex for centration of the multifocal single piece intraocular lens. Can J Ophthalmol. 2011;46(4):319-321. DOI: 10.1016/j.jcjo.2011.06.007

[132] Grzybowski A, Kanclerz P. Early postoperative intraocular pressure elevation following cataract surgery. Curr Opin Ophthalmol. 2019;30(1):56-62. DOI: 10.1097/ICU.0000000000000545

[133] Malyugin B. Review of surgical management of small pupils in cataract surgery: Use of the Malyugin ring. Techn Ophthalmol. 2010;8:104-118. DOI: 10.1097/ITO.0b013e318242c452

[134] Malyugin B. Cataract surgery in small pupils. Indian J Ophthalmol. 2017;65(12):1323-1328. DOI:10.4103/ijo.IJO_800_17

[135] Papaconstantinou D, Kalantzis G, Brouzas D, Kontaxakis A, Koutsandrea C, Diagourtas A, Georgalas I. Safety and efficacy of phacoemulsification and intraocular lens implantation through a small pupil using minimal iris manipulation. Clin Interv Aging. 2016;11:651-657. DOI: 10.2147/CIA.S97254

[136] Bhogal MM, Angunawela RI, Little BC. Use of low-cost video recording device in reflective practice in cataract surgery. J Cataract Refract Surg. 2010;36(4):542-546. DOI: 10.1016/j.jcrs.2009.10.053

[137] Verion Reference Unit. Alcon Laboratories. Fort Worth, Texas. Available from: http://crstoday.com/pdfs/0614_supp2.pdf [Accessed: 2020-12-31].

[138] CALLISTO Eye, Computer assisted cataract surgery, ZEISS. Available from: https://www.zeiss.com/meditec/int/products/ophthalmology-optometry/cataract/visualization/computer-assisted-cataract-surgery/callisto-eye.html#highlights. [Accessed: 2020-12-31].

[139] Alfonso JF, Puchades C, Fernandez-Vega L, Merayo C, Montes-Mico R. Contrast sensitivity comparison between AcrySof ReSTOR and Acri.LISA aspheric intraocular lenses. J Refract Surg. 2010;26:471-477. DOI: 10.3928/1081597X-20090728-04

[140] Alba-Bueno F, Vega F, Millán MS. Halos y lentes intraoculares multifocales: origen e interpretación [Halos and multifocal intraocular lenses: origin and interpretation]. Arch Soc Esp Oftalmol. 2014;89(10):397-404. Spanish. DOI: 10.1016/j.oftal.2014.01.002

[141] Montés-Micó R, España E, Bueno I, Charman WN, Menezo JL. Visual performance with multifocal intraocular lenses: mesopic contrast sensitivity under distance and near conditions. Ophthalmology. 2004;111(1):85-96. DOI: 10.1016/S0161-6420(03)00862-5

[142] Galor A, Gonzalez M, Goldman D, O'Brien TP. Intraocular lens exchange surgery in dissatisfied patients with refractive intraocular lenses. J Cataract Refract Surg 2009;35:1706-1710. DOI: 10.1016/j.jcrs.2009.05.022

[143] Schrecker J, Blass S, Langenbucher A. Silicone-diffractive versus acrylic-refractive supplementary

iols: visual performance and manual handling. J Refract Surg. 2014;30(1):41-48. DOI: 10.3928/1081597x-20131217-05

[144] Cillino S, Casuccio A, Di Pace F, Morreale R, Pillitteri F, Cillino G, Lodato G. One-year outcomes with new-generation multifocal intraocular lenses. Ophthalmology. 2008;115(9):1508-1516. DOI: 10.1016/j.ophtha.2008.04.017

[145] Woodward MA, Randleman JB, Stulting RD. Dissatisfaction after multifocal intraocular lens implantation. J Cataract Refract Surg. 2009;35:992-997. DOI: 10.1016/j.jcrs.2009.01.031

[146] Venter JA, Pelouskova M, Collins BM, Schallhorn SC, Hannan SJ. Visual outcomes and patient satisfaction in 9366 eyes using a refractive segmented multifocal intraocular lens. J Cataract Refract Surg. 2013;39:1477-1484. DOI: 10.1016/j.jcrs.2013.03.035

[147] Fernandez-Buenaga R, Alio JL, Munoz-Negrete FJ, Barraquer Compte RI, Alio-Del Barrio JL. Causes of IOL explantation in Spain. Eur J Ophthalmol. 2012;22:762-768.

[148] Dwayne K. Logan. Halos With Multifocal IOLs. A surgeon explores neuroadaptation to reduce complications with these lenses. Cataract and Refractive Surgery Today. 2008. Available from: https://crstoday.com/articles/2008-sep/crst0908_08-php/ [Accessed: 2021-01-20].

[149] Vega-Estrada A, Alió del Barrio JL, Alió JL. Accommodative Intraocular Lenses. In: Alió JL, Pikkel J, editors. Multifocal Intraocular Lenses. The Art and the Practice. 2nd ed. Switzerland: Springer Nature; 2019. p. 355-366. DOI: 10.1007/978-3-030-21282-7_11

[150] Alió JL, Alió Del Barrio JL, Vega-Estrada A. Accommodative intraocular lenses: where are we and where we are going. Eye Vis (Lond). 2017;4:16. DOI: 10.1186/s40662-017-0077-7

[151] Pepose JS, Burke J, Qazi M. Accommodating Intraocular Lenses. Asia Pac J Ophthalmol (Phila). 2017;6(4):350-357. DOI: 10.22608/APO.2017198

[152] Kanclerz P, Toto F, Grzybowski A, Alio JL. Extended Depth-of-Field Intraocular Lenses: An Update. Asia Pac J Ophthalmol (Phila). 2020;9(3):194-202. DOI:10.1097/APO.0000000000000296

[153] Zvorničanin J, Zvorničanin E. Premium intraocular lenses: The past, present and future. J Curr Ophthalmol. 2018;30(4):287-296. DOI: 10.1016/j.joco.2018.04.003

[154] Breyer DRH, Kaymak H, Ax T, Kretz FTA, Auffarth GU, Hagen PR. Multifocal intraocular lenses and extended depth of focus intraocular lenses. Asia Pac J Ophthalmol (Phila). 2017;6(4):339-349. DOI: 10.22608/APO.2017186

[155] Nakazawa M, Ohtsuki K. Apparent accommodation in pseudophakic eyes after implantation of posterior chamber intraocular lenses: optical analysis. Invest Ophthalmol Vis Sci. 1984;25(12):1458-1460.

[156] Rocha KM. Extended depth of focus IOLs: the next chapter in refractive technology? J Refract Surg. 2017;33:146-149. DOI: 10.3928/1081597X-20170217-01

[157] Kanclerz P, Toto F, Grzybowski A, Alio JL. Extended Depth-of-Field Intraocular Lenses: An Update. Asia Pac J Ophthalmol (Phila). 2020;9(3):194-202. DOI:10.1097/APO.0000000000000296

[158] Gallego AA, Bará S, Jaroszewicz Z, Kolodziejczyk A. Visual Strehl performance of IOL designs with extended depth of focus. Optom Vis Sci. 2012;89(12):1702-1707. DOI: 10.1097/OPX.0b013e3182775e1a

[159] Domínguez-Vicent A, Esteve-Taboada JJ, Del Águila-Carrasco AJ, Monsálvez-Romin D, Montés-Micó R. In vitro optical quality comparison of 2 trifocal intraocular lenses and 1 progressive multifocal intraocular lens. J Cataract Refract Surg. 2016;42(1):138-147. DOI: 10.1016/j.jcrs.2015.06.040

[160] Domínguez-Vicent A, Esteve-Taboada JJ, Del Águila-Carrasco AJ, Ferrer-Blasco T, Montés-Micó R. In vitro optical quality comparison between the Mini WELL Ready progressive multifocal and the TECNIS Symfony. Graefes Arch Clin Exp Ophthalmol. 2016;254(7):1387-1397. DOI: 10.1007/s00417-015-3240-7

[161] Alio JL. Presbyopic lenses: evidence, masquerade news, and fake news. Asia Pac J Ophthalmol (Phila). 2019;8:273-274. DOI: 10.1097/01.APO.0000577792.28242.2d

[162] Böhm M, Petermann K, Hemkeppler E, Kohnen T. Defocus curves of 4 presbyopia-correcting IOL designs: Diffractive panfocal, diffractive trifocal, segmental refractive, and extended-depth-of-focus. J Cataract Refract Surg. 2019;45(11):1625-1636. DOI: 10.1016/j.jcrs.2019.07.014

[163] Kanclerz P, Toto F, Grzybowski A, Alio JL. Extended Depth-of-Field Intraocular Lenses: An Update. Asia Pac J Ophthalmol (Phila). 2020;9(3):194-202. DOI:10.1097/APO.0000000000000296

[164] Akella SS, Juthani VV. Extended depth of focus intraocular lenses for presbyopia. Curr Opin Ophthalmol. 2018;29(4):318-322. DOI: 10.1097/ICU.0000000000000490

[165] Cochener B; Concherto Study Group. Clinical outcomes of a new extended range of vision intraocular lens: International Multicenter Concerto Study. J Cataract Refract Surg. 2016;42:1268-1275.

[166] Gatinel D, Loicq J. Clinically relevant optical properties of bifocal, trifocal, and extended depth of focus intraocular lenses. J Refract Surg 2016; 32:273-280. DOI: 10.3928/1081597X-20160121-07

[167] Studený P, Kacerovský M, Kacerovská J, Gajarová N, Straňák Z. HYBRIDNÍ MONOVISION [HYBRID MONOVISION]. Cesk Slov Oftalmol. 2017 Spring;73(1):13-16. Czech.

[168] Iida Y, Shimizu K, Ito M. Pseudophakic monovision using monofocal and multifocal intraocular lenses: hybrid monovision. J Cataract Refract Surg 2011; 37(11):2001-2005. DOI: 10.1016/j.jcrs.2011.05.032

[169] Yoon SY, Song IS, Kim JY, Kim MJ, Tchah H. Bilateral mix-and-match versus unilateral multifocal intraocular lens implantation: long-term comparison. J Cataract Refract Surg. 2013;39(11):1682-1690. DOI: 10.1016/j.jcrs.2013.04.043

[170] Hütz WW, Bahner K, Röhrig B, Hengerer F. The combination of diffractive and refractive multifocal intraocular lenses to provide full visual function after cataract surgery. Eur J Ophthalmol. 2010;20(2):370-375. DOI: 10.1177/112067211002000217

[171] Gunenc U, Celik L. Long-term experience with mixing and matching refractive array and diffractive CeeOn multifocal intraocular lenses. J Refract Surg. 2008;24(3):233-242. DOI: 10.3928/1081597X-20080301-04

[172] Grzybowski A, Kanclerz P. Do we need day-1 postoperative follow-up after cataract surgery? Graefes Arch Clin Exp Ophthalmol. 2019;257(5):855-861. DOI: 10.1007/s00417-018-04210-0

[173] Buckhurst PJ, Naroo SA, Davies LN, Shah S, Drew T, Wolffsohn JS. Assessment of dysphotopsia in pseudophakic subjects

with multifocal intraocular lenses. BMJ Open Ophthalmol. 2017;1(1):e000064. DOI: 10.1136/bmjophth-2016-000064

[174] Steinberg EP, Tielsch JM, Schein OD, Javitt JC, Sharkey P, Cassard SD, Legro MW, Diener-West M, Bass EB, Damiano AM, Steinwachs DM, Sommer A. The VF-14. an index of functional impairment in patients with cataract. Arch Ophthalmol. 1994;112:630-638. DOI: 10.1001/archopht.1994.01090170074026

[175] Mangione CM, Lee PP, Gutierrez PR, Spritzer K, Berry S, Hays RD; National Eye Institute Visual Function Questionnaire Field Test Investigators. Development of the 25-item National Eye Institute Visual Function Questionnaire. Arch Ophthalmol. 2001;119(7):1050-1058. DOI: 10.1001/archopht.119.7.1050.

[176] Lundström M, Pesudovs K. Catquest-9SF patient outcomes questionnaire: nine-item short-form Rasch-scaled revision of the Catquest questionnaire. J Cataract Refract Surg. 2009;35(3):504-513. DOI: 10.1016/j.jcrs.2008.11.038

[177] Radner W, Willinger U, Obermayer W, Mudrich C, Velikay-Parel M, Eisenwort B. A new reading chart for simultaneous determination of reading vision and reading speed. Klin Monatsbl Augenheilkd. 1998;213(3):174-181. DOI: 10.1055/s-2008-1034969

[178] Mansfield JS, Ahn SJ, Legge GE, Luebker A. A new reading acuity chart for normal and low vision. Opt Soc Am Techn Digest. 1993;3:232-235.

[179] Calabrèse A, To L, He Y, Berkholtz E, Rafian P, Legge GE. Comparing performance on the MNREAD iPad application with the MNREAD acuity chart. J Vis. 2018;18(1):8. DOI: 10.1167/18.1.8.

[180] Labiris G, Panagiotopoulou EK, Chatzimichael E, Tzinava M, Mataftsi A, Delibasis K. Introduction of a digital near-vision reading test for normal and low vision adults: development and validation. Eye Vis (Lond). 2020;7:51. DOI: 10.1186/s40662-020-00216-0

[181] Emily B. Worrall, BS, BA, and Hoon C. Jung, MD. Blended Vision With Multifocal Intraocular Lenses. EyeNet Magazine. American Academy of Ophthslmology. 2019. Available from: https://www.aao.org/eyenet/article/blended-vision-with-multifocal-intraocular-lenses [Accessed: 2021-01-08]

Chapter 7

Successful Premium Multifocal IOL Surgery: Key Issues and Pearls

Chen Xu

Abstract

Premium multifocal IOLs are a popular option for cataract or presbyopia patients today. Patients can achieve high levels of success and satisfaction after these advanced technology IOLs implantation. However, adequate preoperative clinical evaluation including patient selection, optical and anatomical examination is crucial to reach a success case. Based on the preoperative diagnosis including the corneal astigmatism, biometry measurement, IOL power calculation, presbyopia correcting IOLs' indications and contraindications should be assessed for IOL selection strategy. Surgical procedure should be technically optimized to achieve the best outcomes. Adequate management of both satisfied and unsatisfied patients will improve the benefit of current premium IOLs.

Keywords: premium IOL surgery, patient selection

1. Introduction

Premium multifocal intraocular lenses (IOLs) became more and more popular in modern cataract surgery after new millennium year [1, 2]. In tandem, the advances in ophthalmologic surgical approach such as femtosecond laser assisted cataract surgery (FLACS) [3], the improvement in biometry and IOL power calculation [4], the development of the intraocular lens techniques [5] led to successfully correct presbyopia, astigmatism and other refractive error through cataract or lens exchange surgery. These premium IOLs surgeries especially the presbyopia-correcting procedures can offer patients more visual and life quality without spectacle. But there are many key issues in the presbyopia-correcting procedure including proper patient selection, preoperative counseling, surgical planning and techniques which should be focused during perioperative stage.

2. Premium IOLs

Comparing with conventional IOL, premium IOLs can offer more and better visual function. But there are no standard criteria about premium IOL due to the continual evolution of the IOLs' technology. The aspherical IOL, blue light filter IOL, toric IOL had been defined as premium IOLs in the past decades. This chapter will highlight the presbyopia correcting IOLs as the premium IOLs in the following paragraph. The presbyopia correcting IOLs can be classified into three groups: accommodative IOLs, refractive or diffractive multifocal IOLs and extended depth of focus (EDOF) IOLs according to its optical design and physical properties.

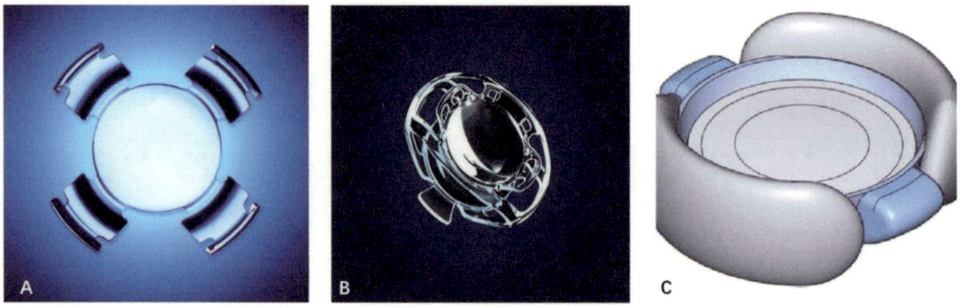

Figure 1.
Accommodating intraocular lenses. (A): 1CU, HumamOptics; (B): Dual-optic synchrony IOL, AMO; (C): FluidVision accommodating IOL, PowerVision.

2.1 Accommodating intraocular lenses

Accommodative IOL are designated to produce a dynamic power with the change of IOL optic position, shape or refractive index by pseudoaccommodating and/or accommodating mechanisms with contraction of the ciliary muscle [6]. There are several accommodative IOLs design strategies: single-optic, dual-optic and deformable optic IOLs (**Figure 1**). Single-optic accommodative IOL (Crystalens, Bausch & Lomb; 1CU, Human Optics) possess the hinge design between the optic and the haptic to facilitate the anterior axial movement of effective lenses position with pressure of the capsule bag and vitreous during the accommodative stimulus. Previous studies demonstrated that 1 mm of optic movement is equivalent of 2 D of power change [7]. But the clinical studies had not demonstrated the consistent accommodation amplitude of the pseudoaccomodating IOL eyes especially in the long term follow up. Dual-optic Synchrony IOL (Abbott Medical Optics, AMO) utilize a positively powered biconvex front lens (+32D) connected to a negatively powered concave-convex lens. During the accommodative effort, the distance between the two optic elements increased that lead to increasing effective power of the overall lens [8]. The deformable optic design IOLs like FluidVision accommodating IOL (PowerVision) still underwent investigation in lab or clinical trial research. Though there are no contrast sensitivity loss or dysphotopsias issue, all these accommodative IOLs still have their limitations about the inability to consistently generate large amounts of accommodative power.

2.2 Multifocal IOL

There are two type multifocal IOLs according to optical design principle: refractive and diffractive IOLs (**Figure 2**).

Refractive multifocal IOLs based on the different dioptic power zone with the light ray's refraction principles. These zones provide various focal points, allowing for an improvement in distance, intermediate, and near vision. Though refractive multifocal IOL can afford good quality vision, the limitation of these symmetric multifocal lens (Array, Abbott Medical Optics; ReZoom, Abbott Medical Optics) are pupillary size and lens centration dependence. The asymmetric segmental refractive IOLs (Lentis Mplus, Oculentis) has been intended to reduce this problem and available for patients with low acceptance for dysphotopsia [9].

Diffractive multifocal IOLs rely on concentric diffractive surfaces on the optic portion of the lens, this causes constructive and destructive interference of optic wavefronts to provide two or three focality which led to bifocal or trifocal IOLs. A different approach about diffractive ring pattern, diffractive ring width and

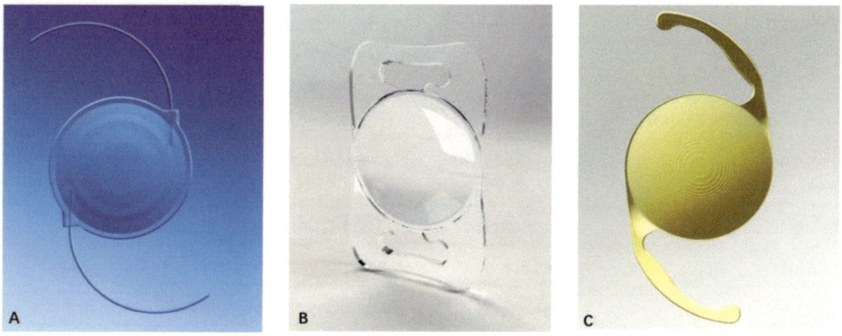

Figure 2.
Multifocal IOL. (A): Array IOL, AMO; (B): Lentis Mplus IOL, Oculentis; (C): ReSTOR IOL, Alcon.

step height by different manufactures introduces different add power and light distribution. Larger ring width provides less addition power and small ring width provides more addition power, while higher steps sends more light to distant focal point and lower step sends more lights to near focal point. The IOL (Restor, Alcon) with refractive-diffractive mix pattern and apodized steps which has concentric rings of decreasing height intends to influence light distribution between distant and near focal points on pupil size [10]. Multifocal IOLs are associated with higher rates of spectacle independence than monofocal IOLs, but are more frequently associated with dysphotopsias and decreased contrast sensitivity [2].

2.3 Extended depth of focus IOLs

Extended depth of focus (EDOF) IOLs are a newer category of IOLs that aims to give an elongated focus of vision, that enhances depth of focus rather than introduces several foci. It can reduce photic phenomena, glare, and halos, which have been reported in traditional multifocal IOLs. Tecnis Symfony IOL (Abbott Medical Optics) was the first EDOF IOL approved in 2016 by the U.S. Food and Drug Administration (FDA) (**Figure 3**). Now, there are several EDOF IOLs had been released in the market which had combined with different techniques such as diffractive optical design, spherical aberration, chromatic aberration, pinhole effect [11]. American Academy of Ophthalmology has provided consensus

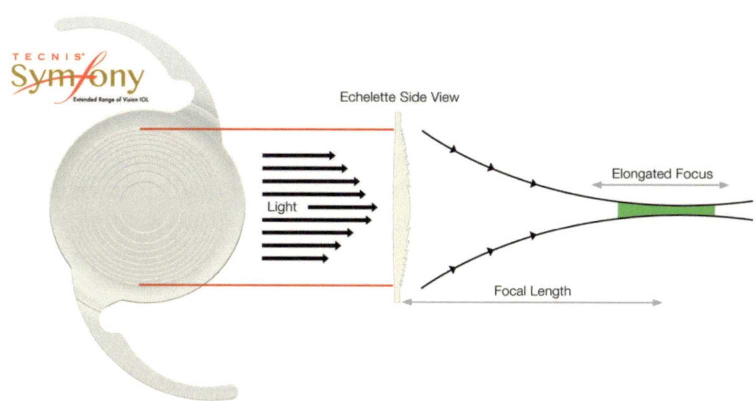

Figure 3.
EDOF IOLs: Symfony IOL.

Premium IOL	Principle	Optical design	Focality	Interm/ Near Add(D)
Crystalens (Bausch & Lomb)	Accommodative	Single-Optics	Accommodating	>0.4
1CU (Human Optics)	Accommodative	Single-Optics	Accommodating	1.36 ~ 2.25 [15]
Synchrony IOLs (AMO)	Accommodative	Duel-Optics	Accommodating	1
Array (AMO)	Refractive	Zonal, progressive	2	0/3.5
ReZoom (AMO)	Refractive	Zonal,progressive	2	0/3.5
Restor (+4,+3,+2.5) (Alcon)	Diffractive	Symmetric, Apodized	2	0/4.0 0/3.0 0/2.5
Tecnis ZKB, ZLB, ZMB (AMO)	Diffractive	Symmetric, Constant	2	0/2.75, 0/3.25, 0/4.0
AT Lisa 809MP (Zeiss)	Diffractive	Symmetric, Constant	2	0/3.75
SBL 2 and 3 (Lenstec INC)	Refractive	Asymmetric. Segmental	2	0/2, 0/3
Mplus Lentis MF 20/30(X) (Oculentis)	Refractive	Asymmetric. Segmental	2	0/2, 0/3
PanOptix AcrySof (Alcon)	Diffractive	Diffractive, Constant	3	2.17/3.25
AT Lisa Tri (Zeiss)	Diffractive	Diffractive, Zone	3	1.67/3.3
FineVision (PhysIOL)	Diffractive	Apodized Diffractive	3	1.75/3.5
Comfort Lentis MF 15 (Oculentis)	EDOF	Refractive	2	1.5/0
Symfony Tecnis (AMO)	EDOF	Diffractive, achromate	EDOF	1.75/0
Mini Well Ready (Sifi Meditec)	EDOF	Progressive, Spherical aberration	EDOF	0/3
IC-8 (AcuFocus)	EDOF	Masked, Pin-hole	EDOF	

Table 1.
Properties of popular premium intraocular lenses (IOLs) [10, 11].

statement for EDOF IOL. These should have an extended far focus area which reaches the intermediate distance, providing excellent intermediate vision. Depth of focus should be at least 0.5 D wider than monofocal IOL for distance visual acuity of 0.03 logMAR [12]. Nevertheless, in practice, EDOF lenses provide excellent intermediate vision, but inadequate quality of vision for near distance [13, 14] (**Table 1**).

3. Patients selection

Even the IOLs technique progress offers patients the possibility of spectacle independence, the selection of presbyopia correction candidates is the most important issue which can lead to a successful surgery [16]. The right patients are the cataract or presbyopia patients who seek an intraocular IOLs solution to spectacle independence. The surgeon should understand patient's expectations about visual task. A detailed discussion should be held to explain the limitations of premium IOLs to patient, that can establish their realistic expectation [17].

The characteristics of lifestyle or work is also an important selection criterion for premium IOL procedure. Ophthalmologists choose the correct type multifocal IOLs depending on what they do or where they live. Different cultures expressed different visual requirement on lifestyle and work. There may be a lot of time-consuming on near work with the computer, tablet, mobile phone, and on near life with book reading in Asian people, while there are more of an outdoor life in western populations. Especially, Chinese text may be very small and intricate comparing to English character, and hence a full reading add is usually needed. Furthermore, Asian people are generally shorter figure and shorter arms which cause the shorter distance between the face and the book, the mobile phone and other materials. Low add multifocal IOLs or normal monovision strategies may not be able to cope with the demands of reading in Asian people. The near vision satisfaction will be gain better in western population than Asian people. When such near vision is a high priority, high add multifocal IOLs or full-range multifocal IOL is the better solution.

Age also plays an important role in patient selection. Several conditions become more prevalent with age, such as optic neuropathy, macular degeneration and ocular surface disease, that may compound the loss of contrast sensitivity seen in multifocal IOLs. The examination of ocular disease using OCT, visual field, visual electrophysiology will provide some information about the post-operative visual quality results. These age-related diseases will be discussion in below. Multifocal IOLs implantation in pediatric cataract case is the subject of much controversy [18]. Amblyopia is common in these patients especially in unilateral pediatric cataract patients, while multifocal IOLs will reduce the contrast sensitivity and exacerbate amblyopia. Another issue is the ongoing growing of the child resulting in the question of how to calculate the power of the implanted lens, because the target refractive status depend on the age of the patient and the visual demands. There are just a few publications on this subject, we also did not have any experiences of multifocal IOLs in children [19–21].

Patients' current visual acuity and refractive error and should be considered. Hyperopes who have significant cataracts will gain the most from presbyopia correcting IOLs, with uncorrected vision improvement at all distances. Mild myopes who have transparent crystalline lens may be dissatisfied with the result, because they often rely on their near vision for specific tasks and may have something to lose postoperatively.

Before choosing the presbyopia correcting IOLs, the surgeon should spend a lot of time in counseling with patients to access the personality, occupation and lifestyle of patients. In some clinics, a questionnaire is also helpful for evaluating patient's needs and ranking patient's personality from "easygoing" to "perfectionist" (**Figure 4**). It is important to rule out those patients who have unreasonable expectations about perfect visual needs or who have anxiety, doubt, nervousness characteristics. Those patients are more likely to be dissatisfied with presbyopia correcting IOLs. A visual behavior monitor that patients can wear on their spectacles to track their visual behavior and environment, now provides a lifestyle match index to help ophthalmologist convert that data into useful clinical information to select the best IOL for a given patient [22].

Some patients who need the specific vision requirement in their daily work and life also should be excluded out of the candidate, such as airline pilots, truck drivers, taxi drivers and anyone whose job requires activity at night or low-light conditions. The patients who often mention halos and glare disturb their jobs also should

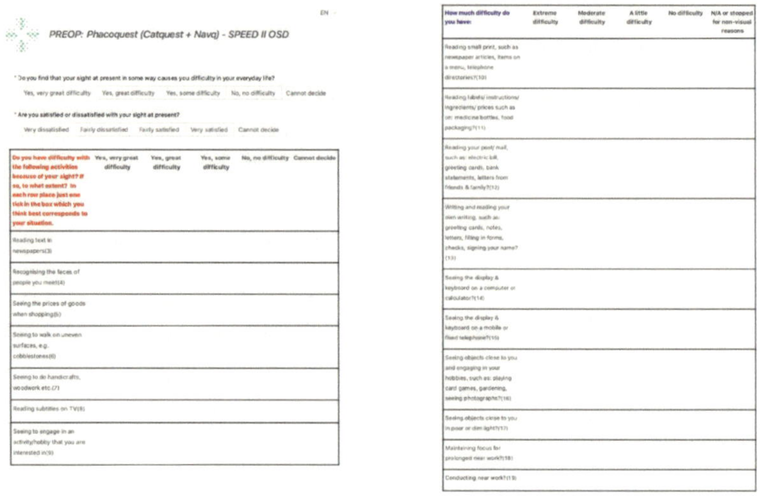

EN

PREOP: Phacoquest (Catquest + Navq) - SPEED II OSD

* Do you find that your sight at present in some way causes you difficulty in your everyday life?

Yes, very great difficulty | Yes, great difficulty | Yes, some difficulty | No, no difficulty | Cannot decide

* Are you satisfied or dissatisfied with your sight at present?

Very dissatisfied | Fairly dissatisfied | Fairly satisfied | Very satisfied | Cannot decide

Do you have difficulty with the following activities because of your sight? If so, to what extent? In each row place just one tick in the box which you think best corresponds to your situation.	Yes, very great difficulty	Yes, great difficulty	Yes, some difficulty	No, no difficulty	Cannot decide
Reading text in newspapers(3)					
Recognising the faces of people you meet(4)					
Seeing the prices of goods when shopping(5)					
Seeing to walk on uneven surfaces, e.g. cobblestones(6)					
Seeing to do handicrafts, woodwork etc.(7)					
Reading subtitles on TV(8)					
Seeing to engage in an activity/hobby that you are interested in(9)					

How much difficulty do you have:	Extreme difficulty	Moderate difficulty	A little difficulty	No difficulty	N/A or stopped for non-visual reasons
Reading small print, such as newspaper articles, items on a menu, telephone directories?(10)					
Reading labels/ instructions/ ingredients/ prices such as on: medicine bottles, food packaging?(11)					
Reading your post/ mail, such as: electric bill, greeting cards, bank statements, letters from friends & family?(12)					
Writing and reading your own writing, such as: greeting cards, notes, letters, filling in forms, checks, signing your name?(13)					
Seeing the display & keyboard on a computer or calculator?(14)					
Seeing the display & keyboard on a mobile or fixed telephone?(15)					
Seeing objects close to you and engaging in your hobbies, such as: playing card games, gardening, seeing photographs?(16)					
Seeing objects close to you in poor or dim light?(17)					
Maintaining focus for prolonged near work?(18)					
Conducting near work?(19)					

Figure 4.
Preoperative questionnaire (courtesy of dr. Takashi).

be rule out of the candidates. The diffractive or refractive multifocal IOLs will increased the photic phenomena in dim environment, while the accommodation IOL or monovision based on the monofocal IOLs should be better choice.

4. Preoperative ocular evaluation

The detailed preoperative examination of clinical ophthalmologic conditions should be done to help patients achieve good results because a successful presbyopia correcting solution often based on a health eye. Choosing the right presbyopia correcting IOLs should be considered for biometry, keratometry, topography and pupil reactivity and other eye comorbidities.

4.1 Corneal astigmatism

It is important to correct astigmatism in the premium IOLs surgery. The postoperative astigmatism should be less than 0.75D in the eye which bifocal or trifocal IOL had been implanted. Over 1.5 diopter postoperative astigmatism is one of main reasons for patient's dissatisfaction following surgery. The larger amounts of postoperative astigmatism will cause decreasing visual function of multifocal IOLs, increasing some optical phenomena [23].

The keratometry, autorefraction and corneal topography/tomography are the helpful preoperative diagnostic devices to evaluate patients with astigmatism to select the astigmatism correction option——limbal relaxing incisions (LRI) or toric presbyopia correcting IOLs. The corneal topography provides more detailed useful information on the regularity of the corneal astigmatism than conventional keratometry or optical biometry (IOLMaster, Lenstar). Tomography devices like Pentacam address the posterior corneal astigmatism or total corneal astigmatism which deliver to more accuracy correcting astigmatism in multifocal IOLs cases (**Figure 5**). Another important issue in management of corneal astigmatism is surgical induced astigmatism which results from flattening in the meridian of the incision and steepening 90° away. The surgeon should evaluate his surgical induced astigmatism (SIA) via standard astigmatic vector analysis or online calculator [24].

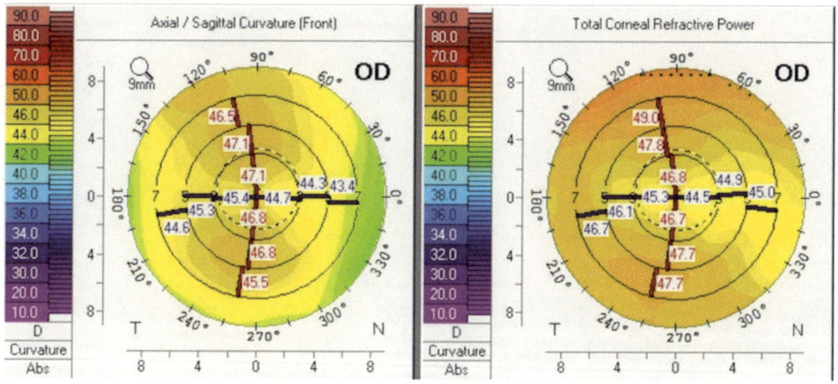

Figure 5.
Regular corneal astigmatism and total corneal astigmatism.

Small amounts of regular astigmatism can be corrected with manual LRI or femtosecond laser LRI, the later method achieved a higher correction and lower postoperative cylinder than manual LRI patients [25]. LRI correction is determined by Abbott Medical Optics' LRI calculator (http://www.lricalculator.com).

The toric presbyopia correcting IOLs is more predictable treatment than LRI, providing good uncorrected vision at distance and either intermediate or near, depending on the built-in add [26, 27]. The toric IOL can be calculated with online program provided by the IOL manufacturer. Most of online calculators had taken into consideration anterior corneal astigmatism, posterior corneal astigmatism and SIA, and choosing IOL toricity by using the total corneal refractive power or in-built nomogram. Some new technologies had been developed to improve toric multifocal IOLs solution flow to achieve the better outcome, including intraoperative wavefront aberrometry (ORA system, Alcon), Image Guided System like Verion(Alcon), Callisto Eye (Carl Zeiss Meditec).

Corneal with irregular astigmatism is contraindicator for multifocal IOLs. Irregular astigmatism often caused by previous corneal infection disease, trauma, dystrophies, pterygium or severe dry eye. In these conditions, poor higher-order root-mean square (HO RMS) corneal wavefront error over a 6-mm zone will present in Pentacam or other aberrometry. If this value exceeds 0.50 μm, the patient will have a high risk of halos and glare with a multifocal IOL (**Figure 6**).

4.2 Keratoconus

Cataract surgery in keratoconic eyes is not uncommon issue which need to be addressed. Proper IOL selection must be individualized for each keratoconic patient to achieve an optimal outcome. Even for monofocal IOLs implantation, IOLs power calculation is a challenging issue due to the abnormalities of both anterior and posterior corneal surface [28]. Some studies have shown promising results about toric IOL in nonprogress keratoconic patients, while in progress cases the combined procedures including intracorneal ring segment (ICRS), cross linking and toric IOL is preferred [29, 30].

But multifocal IOLs should been avoided because the loss of contrast sensitivity associated with multifocal lenses will be magnified by the corneal irregularity. Previous corneal surgical history like pterygium, PKP is an important etiology for irregular astigmatism. IOL solution in these cases is similar to the keratoconus cases.

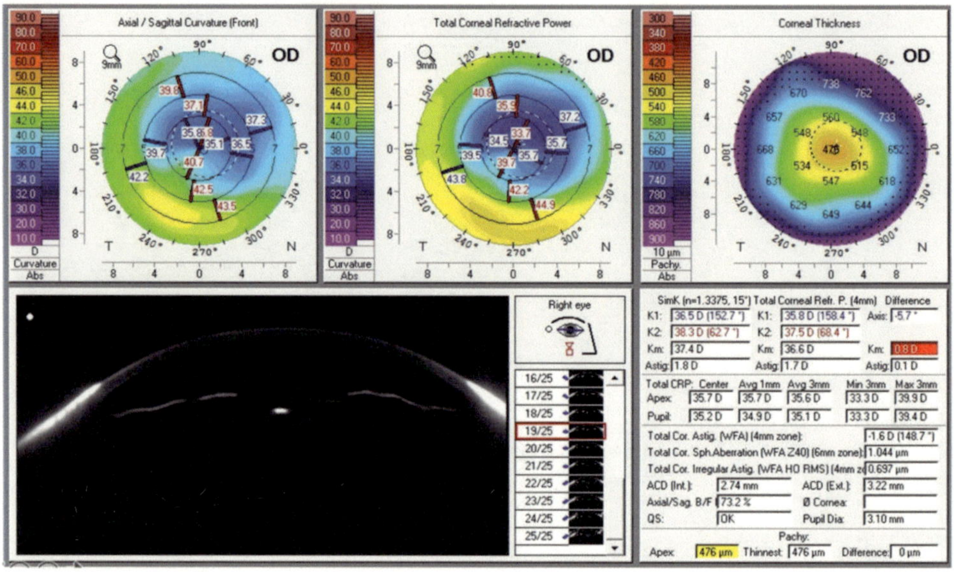

Figure 6.
Corneal irregular astigmatism with history of corneal refractive surgery. HO RMS is 0.679 um, over 0.50 um.

4.3 Previous corneal refractive surgery

Patients who have undergone myopic or hyperopic LASIK/PRK/RK tend to select the premium IOLs with higher expectations regarding the refractive outcome. But intraocular lens power calculation for these patients is challenging because it is difficult to calculate the true corneal power. The optical quality of corneal is another factor to consider for IOL selection. The high order aberration is increased after the laser myopic corneal which led to decrease the visual result of multifocal IOLs and increase the photophobia like halo, glare [31]. If cornea high order aberration is higher than 1 μm especially it caused by corneal irregularities, the presence of irregular astigmatism/coma, a decentered/uneven treatment bed, the patient should not be considered as good candidate for multifocal IOL implantation [5].

The post-myopic LASIK patients who had previous treatment was less then −6 D, ablation bed was fairly well centered with no or little irregular astigmatism and did not experience problems with night vision can be considered to use presbyopia correcting IOLs. [32] Some surgeon preferred EDOF IOls (Symfony, Johnson and Johnson Vision) in these patients, because its larger size central optic and higher light transmission provides an enhanced contrast sensitivity as compared with other refractive or diffractive multifocal IOls [33, 34]. If monovision was already created with LASIK or PRK, and monovision is probably a much better way to go.

In the patients who had underwent the hyperopia laser correctio have increased negative spherical aberration and are best suited for aberration-free multifocal IOLs or IOLs with positive spherical aberration. The accommodating IOL was recommend by some surgeon if multifocal IOLs and EDOF IOLs were intolerant by the significant corneal coma.

A monofocal IOL is often the best choice in patients with previous RK who often had irregular corneal or increased corneal aberration. Now, pinhole IOLs (Xtrafocus, Morcher GmbH) is an effective presbyopia correcting solution for irregular astigmatism RK patients. It can correct of postoperative residual refraction and provide an elongated depth of focus [35].

4.4 Ocular surface disease (OSD)

Understanding the patient's ocular surface is of critical importance because ocular surface pathologic features can lead to false corneal power, induced astigmatism and unstable bad visual acuity.

Preoperative dry eye will lead to post-operative refractive surprise, blur vision and foreign body sensation, excessive tearing, and photophobia that makes patients unhappy [36]. Surgeon and assistor should address the OSD issue as part of preoperative discussion to management the patient expectation.

The most common OSD is meibomian gland dysfunction and dye eye. A thorough evaluation of the lids and lashes, testing for lacrimal gland function and tear film should be included in preoperative examination. A symptoms questionnaire also helps to capture OSD before surgery.

The treatment is based on severity and subtype of OSD. Steroid and preservative-free lubrication can be used for improving the corneal surface. Other therapy included moisture chamber glass, punctal occlusion, and oral omega fatty acid supplements. If the ocular surface condition is not improved after advanced therapies, the multifocal IOLs is not recommend due to significantly high and persistent postoperative OSD symptoms [37]. The low tear breakup time, increased meibomian gland dropout will increase the high order aberration leading to decrease the visual quality after the premium IOLs implantation [16].

Besides OSD, there are some corneal disease inducing irregular astigmatism will affect the premium IOLs section, such as addressing anterior basement membrane dystrophy (ABMD), epithelial basement membrane dystrophy, Salzmann nodular degeneration (SND). Appropriate management of these corneal abnormalities should be performed before cataract surgery in order to gain the reliable corneal keratometry and other ocular biometry parameter.

4.5 Pupil size, angle kappa and angle alpha

Pupil size, shape and centration also have a significant influence on presbyopic IOL surgery. In diffractive multifocal IOLs, the difference of diffractive step height determined the different light energy distribution in far, intermediate and near distance. Light energy distribution of the multifocal IOLs (MIOLs) varies with different aperture. For apodized diffractive IOLs, the near reading will become difficulty due to light energy goes more to distance in dim illumination. It suggested eyes implanted with multifocal IOLs should have a photopic pupil size of 3.5 mm or less and mesopic pupil size of 5 mm or less [38]. The average pupil size of photopic and mesopic are correlated with contrast sensitivity defocus curve [38]. The photophobia phenomenon like glare and halo also more complained in the large pupil patients. For the asymmetric refractive multifocal IOLs, the pupil size is an important parameter which had a significant negative subjective impact for outcomes [39].

Angle kappa (K) is defined as the angular difference between the visual axis and the pupillary axis while angle a refers to the angular distance between the visual axis and the optical axis. Though postoperative far, intermediate, and near vision is not affected by angle K which does not include the fixation point, large angle K might play a role in the decentration of multifocal intraocular lenses (IOLs), potentially resulting in the incident of glare and hola increasing which led to patient satisfaction with multifocal IOLs [40–43]. A well-centered lens in the visual axis is vital for proper functioning of presbyopic IOLs. Chord between the pupil centration and visual axis is the value to be evaluated for IOL location. It was suggested that a MIOL is unacceptable for use if the k value is greater than half of the diameter of

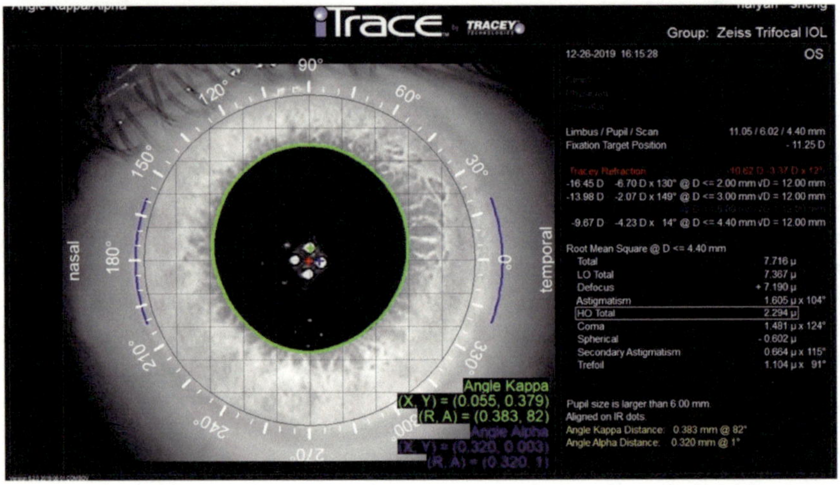

Figure 7.
Pupil size, angle kappa and angle alpha.

the central optical zone. The limitation of k value is different according to the different multifocal IOLs——ReSTOR(Alcon) 0.4 mm, Tecnis multifocal IOL (Abbott Medical Optics) 0.5 mm, FineVision POD F IOL(PhysIOL) 0.6 mm [44].

Angle alpha is defined by the radial distance between the center of the limbus and the visual axis, which was found to predict the tilt of the IOL in respect to the visual axis. Wang had demonstrated that angle alpha was relatively stable whereas angle kappa changes from pre- to postoperative situation [45]. Angle alpha seems to be a better predictor for photic phenomena and patient satisfaction with multifocal IOLs [46]. But there still was different aspects on the predictive capacity of angle α on the outcome with multifocal IOLs. Piracha had concluded the angle alpha distance is larger than 0.5 mm, the eye is not suitable for multifocal IOL implantation [47], while Fu found there was no statistically significant correlation between angle alpha and the objective visual quality parameters [41] (**Figure** 7).

4.6 Glaucoma

Glaucoma patients often presented with the visual field damage, contrast sensitivity loss, small pupils and capsular and zonular issues, to affect vision outcomes must be taken into account when choosing a premium IOL.

Previous generation multifocal IOLs (Restor, Alcon; ReZoom, Abbott Medical Optics) were reported to significantly reduce the contrast sensitivity, especially in refractive multifocal IOL implantation. New advanced technology multifocal IOL or EDOF IOLs seem to mitigate the loss of contrast sensitivity [48]. And multifocal IOL also affect the visual field test and oct scan in the glaucoma patients' follow-up.

But because of a lack of scientific evidence in the form of large trials on the impact of multifocal IOLs in glaucoma, decisions regarding the implantation in a glaucoma patient should be tailored according to the patient' s motivation and the rate of glaucoma progression. The patient who is glaucoma suspect, ocular hypertensive, early stage with controlled and stable visual field damage is the candidate for diffractive multifocal IOLs and EDOF IOLs. The patients with severe, advanced, progressive glaucoma, or with high risk of pupil or zonular changes like chronic miotics, pseudoexfoliation, pigment dispersion will not benefit of multifocality [49].

4.7 Retinal disease

It is a controversial topic of premium IOLs application in retinal disease patients because there are varying degrees of macular lesion, ranging from drusen without visual damage to the late stages of atrophic AMD. Multifocal IOLs are strictly not recommend in retinitis pigmentosa and Stargardt's disease, while diabetic retinopathy, age-related macular degeneration, and epiretinal membranes are relative contraindications [50]. Beside the different character of retinal diseases, the progression is an important issue to consider for premium IOLs solution [17].

For the mild or stable disease, multifocal IOLs is option for patient with careful and thoroughly consent about the prognosis including the issue of lower contrast sensitivity and long-term results with the disease progressing. Many studies had demonstrated the contrast sensitivity decreased in multifocal IOLs. Due to loss of contrast sensitivity at lower spatial frequencies is also presented even in mild forms of AMD, the EDOF IOLs is preferred in these cases. Multifocal IOLs generally are disadvised for patients with severe AMD because pre-existing pathologic features are a contraindication.

The presence of an epiretinal membrane (ERM) can lead to more unpredictability with the spherical power of the IOL selection and its refractive outcome. Multifocal IOLs in ERM patients will face to the loss of contrast sensitivity, increased risk for postoperative cystoid macular edema [51].

There are few studies addressing the multifocal IOLs and retinal disease, which report a significant improvement in visual-related outcomes than the monofocal implantation. Nevertheless, more research is needed to address the aforementioned concerns and to optimize the use of MIOLs in eyes with retinal disease.

5. Ocular biometry and IOL power calculation

Accurate measurements are critical for determining the correct power of a premium IOL before it is implanted during cataract surgery. The emmetropia is key factor of a successful refractive lens exchange to gain spectacle independence. Attaining this goal requires eliminating astigmatism and achieving a precise postoperative plano refraction within ±0.25 D.

Ocular biometry involves anatomical measurements of the eye, including the axial length (AL), keratometry, anterior chamber depth (ACD), lens thickness (LT), horizonal white to white (HWTW) which are the parameters for IOL power calculation [52].

Even the ultrasound biometry is still used in some difficult cases such as brunescent cataract, white cataract and severe subcapsular cataract. A hyperopic surprise often appeared in high myopic patients by using ultrasound biometry, because A-scan measured the deepest part of the staphyloma while macula was on the edge of the staphyloma which led to false longer axial length.

With IOLMaster (Zeiss) introduced in 1999, optical biometry technique provide a directly measurement from the macula to the corneal vertex. It becomes golden standard as it is highly accurate, easy to perform, non-invasive and comfortable for the patient. The accuracy of optical biometry, and in particular the IOLMaster 500 (Zeiss) and Lenstar 900 (Haag-Streit), have been extensively confirmed across a wide range of scientific studies [53, 54]. New generational optical biometry IOLMaster 700 (Zeiss) has integrate swept source optical coherence tomography to measure axial length. It allows for penetration of dense cataracts, determination of lens thickness (not available on the prior generations of IOLmaster), and visualization of the foveal pit to both ensure alignment of the image and possibly detect pathology like epiretinal membrane or cystoid macular edema which is influenced the premium IOLs power calculation [55].

Besides the accuracy biometry, the IOL power calculation formula choice also is critical for premium IOLs surgery. Though the third and newer generation formula can get accuracy refractive result in normal axis length and keratometry eyes, attention must be paid to the long axial length eye as well as the abnormal corneal power cases [56]. New IOL power calculation formula like Barrett, Hill-RBF and Olsen will achieve more precision and accuracy in longer and short axial length eyes [57].

The IOL power calculation in post corneal refractive surgery eyes always is a challenge issue. Whether corneal radical keratotomy or PRK/LASIK always change the corneal shape of in different ways. Errors in evaluation of the correct corneal power and errors in estimating the effective lens position with the classical thin-lens formulas lead to underestimate the IOL power and hyperopic postoperative refractive surprise. Many adjustment methods had been developed to estimate the true corneal keratometric data such as Haigis-L formula, Shammas no-history formula [58]. The new device like schiempflug or swept source OCT which can directly measure the anterior/posterior/total corneal power to obtain more accuracy results [59]. Modern IOL formulas, such as the Barrett True-K and ascrs.org web-based IOL power calculator can provide greater refractive predictability [60].

Cataract surgeon must personalize his IOL constants for premium lenses. Although the design of the IOL is the primary factor in the constant, variations in surgical technique such as the placement of the IOL, the location and design of the incision, and differences in biometry and technicians also affect the personalized lens constant. Preoperative biometric data and post-operative refractive error of 20 to 40 cases should be collected in order to personalize lens constant [52]. This process is the only way to achieve superior results with these IOLs and accuracy to within ±0.25 D for 95 percent of patients. Personalizing the lens constant is critical to eliminating the systematic variations that make excellent results and happy patients the rule with multifocal lenses.

6. Advanced technology IOL selection strategy

When the patient and ocular conditions had been fully evaluated, the surgeon can match the right advanced technology IOL to the right patients that can ensure positive outcomes. Here we present a premium IOLs decision flowchart based on the detail recommendations mentioned above.

- Patients selection:
    - A strong desire to be independent with spectacle for near, intermediate, far distance
    - A positive attitude and leading an active life, not a perfectionist
    - A job not to require activity at night or low-light condition
- Ocular Feature Checklist
    - Preoperative visual acuity and refractive error
        1. Hyperopic, high myopia and plano presbyopia are good candidates for presbyopia correcting IOL surgery.

ii. Mild myopia with presbyopia patients are typically accustomed to removing their glasses at near, so it is important to set proper expectations

iii. Thorough education and careful counsel are needed for mild myopic patients before presbyopia correcting IOLs surgery.

- Corneal conditions

  i. Dry eye or OSD evaluation and management

  ii. Corneal astigmatism or aberration measurement by using multi-device

  iii. Address the posterior surface corneal astigmatism

  iv. Consider surgical induced astigmatism

- Pupil size and centration

  i. photopic pupil size of 3.5 mm or less and mesopic pupil size of 5 mm or less

  ii. angle Kappa greater than half of the diameter of the central optical zone

- Comorbidities

  i. Post-corneal refractive surgery

  ii. Glaucoma

  iii. Retinal disease

- Biometry measurement and IOL calculation

1. Optical biometry is recommended, which included partial poherence interferometry (PCI) IOLMaster 500, optical low coherence reflectometry Lenstar 900 and SWEPT source OCT IOLMaster 700

2. 3rd and new generation formulal: [61]

   - Haigis, Hoffer Q, Holladay 1 and 2 and SRK/T.

   - Barrett Universal II formula

   - Emmetropia Verifying Optical (EVO), Kane, Næser 2, Olsen, the Panacea, Pearl DGS, Radial Basis Function (RBF), T2 and VRF formulas

3. Special attention to post-refractive surgery IOL calculation issue

- IOLs solutions

Monofocal aspheric IOLs is most common IOLs in modern phacoemulsification surgery which can neutralize the residual corneal spherical aberration and improve contrast sensitivity especially in dim light condition. For the patients with

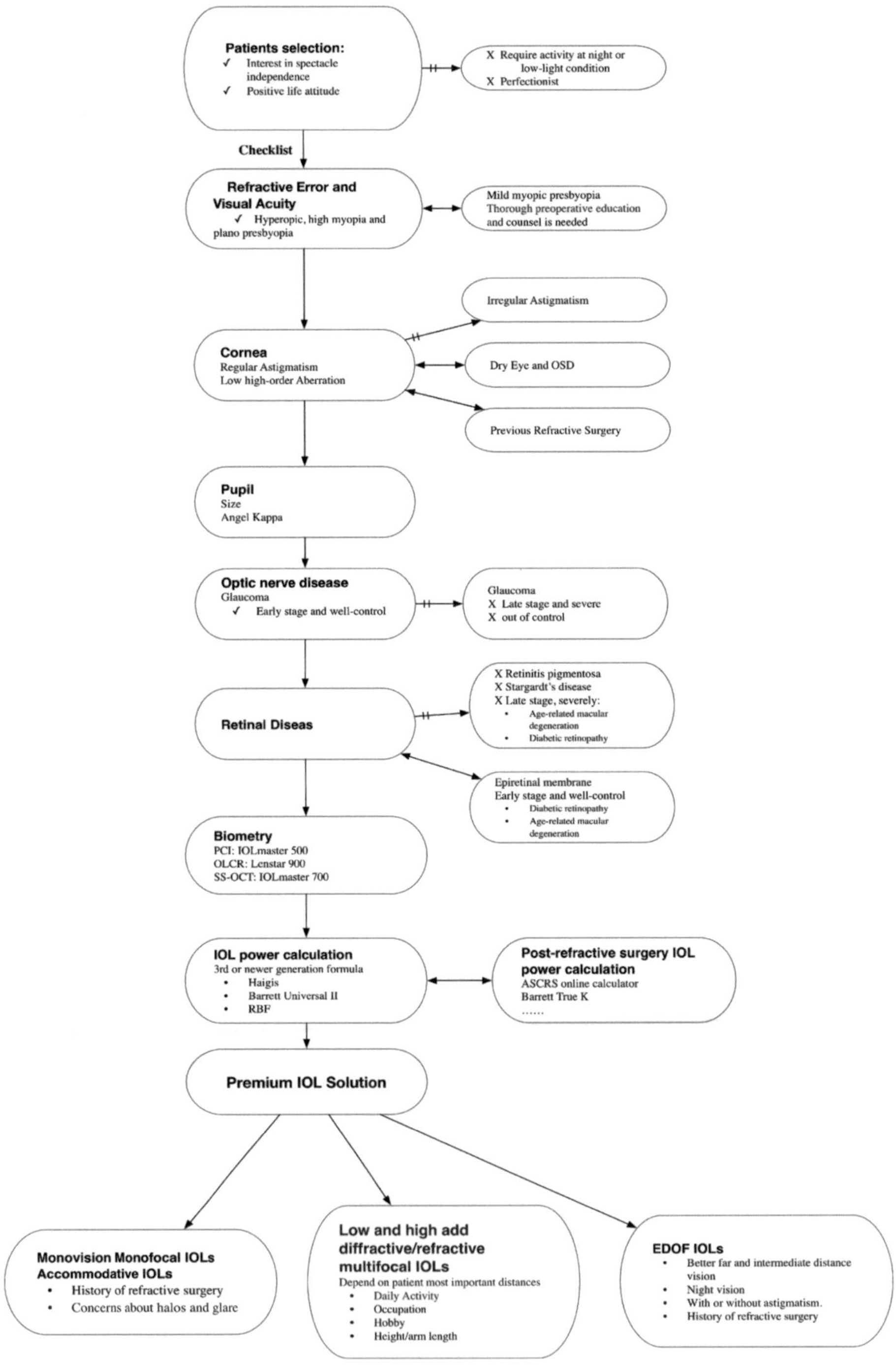

Figure 8.
Flow chart for advanced technology IOL selection.

previous corneal myopic or hyperopic correction procedure or with high concern about halo, glare and night vision, the choice of aspherical IOLs should be tailored basing on the high aberration. Monofocal aspheric IOLs can used for monovision that is a simple solution for presbyopia correcting. It provides monofocal quality of vision, and many patients have been satisfied with this option. However, some patients have reported reduced depth perception, a feeling of imbalance, and limited intermediate vision. There are some modified strategies as mini-monovision or micro monovision which the non-dominant eye targeted for − 0.75 to − 1.25 D (mini-monovision) or around −0.50D (micro-monovision) of myopia to increase visual function at near and intermediate distance [62]. But monovision design may cause some potential problems such as loss of depth perception [63, 64]. A soft contact lens trial is a good predictor for simulating monovision solution, but due to cataract patients often being with worse vision, it is not always indicative of actual visual performance after cataract surgery.

Accommodating IOL is designed for allowing the IOL to move anteriorly or posteriorly, depending on the accommodative forces of the eye. It has the better contrast sensitivity and low photophobia than multifocal IOLs. However, most patients cannot achieve sufficient accommodation for functional near vision and might require reading glasses.

Multifocal IOLs by using refractive or/and diffractive optics is most popular presbyopia correcting IOLs solution in recent years. These type IOLs provide the high patient satisfaction and a better chance of spectacle independence in the refractive lens exchange procedure. Near addition powers are different in different multifocal IOLs, which is often from 1.5D to 4.0D. The higher add can offer a better near vision, but easy led to adverse effects such as dysphotopsia and a reduction in contrast sensitivity. In some aged patients, it will cost several months to neuroadapt of the multifoci images in the retina. To decide which near add power is right for a given patient, the surgeon must evaluate subjective factors (occupations, hobbies, expectations, concernabout night vision) and objective factors (preoperative visual acuity and refraction error, height/arm length).

Extended depth of focus (EDOF) IOLs are a set of intraocular lenses that extend vision instead of offering discrete close, intermediate, or distance vision. These IOLs based on diffractive, pin-hole or aberration technique, while minimizing the quality of vision compromises and night vision symptoms that are associated with multifocal lenses. The EDOF IOLs are more tolerance higher levels of cylinder error, especially for higher amounts of astigmatism in the range of 0.75D to more than 1.0D. Due to EDOF IOLs delivers less spectacle independence than trifocal IOLs, mini-monovision is common strategy with EDOF IOLs implantation. It set the nondominant eye's target at −0.75D, which relates to an extension of the depth of focus, giving the patient the ability to read at a distance of about 45- to-50 cm, thus optimizing their potential for spectacle independence [50]. EDOF IOLs also can be considered for patients who had history of corneal refractive surgery [34] (**Figure 8**).

7. Surgical techniques

Success in cataract surgery with premium IOLs lies in performing every step precisely and predictably. The surgeon team should check the patient's information, the surgical device and material availability.

Surgeons must pay attention to preexisting or surgically induced astigmatism, because it can have a huge impact on visual outcomes with a multifocal IOL. The magnitude of astigmatism and axis should be checked by more than two device such as topography, IOLMaster, Lenstar and so on. For less than 1.0D astigmatism, the incision at steep axis is the better approach. When preoperative astigmatism is up to1.5 diopter, the limbal relaxing incisions (LRIs) can be considerable [65]. At higher levels of astigmatism than 1.5D, the best solution is toric multifocal IOLs [66]. Whether LRI or toric IOLs, the corneal limbal mark should be made before surgery. Many manual method or device had been developed, and computerized automated axis marking system also can been chosen [67].

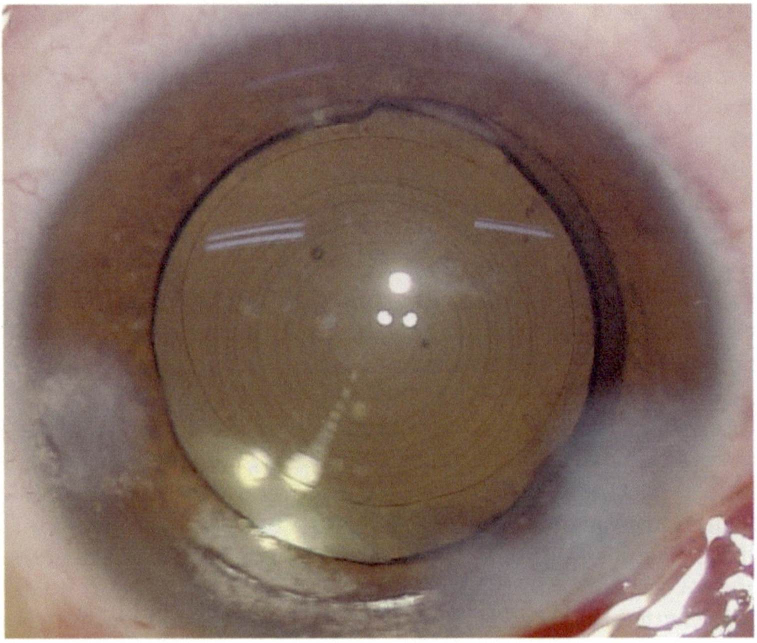

Figure 9.
Trifocal IOL (Panoptix, Alcon) implantation with 5.0 mm FLACS capsulotomy.

A 5.0–5.5 mm perfectly round and centered capsulorhexis is preferred for premium IOLs surgery. The right size capsulorhexis will completely cover the optic of IOLs, let the lens center over the visual axis to get the best visual results. The capsulorhexis size depends on the different IOLs design. The precise size will be customed when femtosecond laser is available, which led to less intraocular aberration postoperatively [68, 69] (**Figure 9**).

The Healon or other viscous ophthalmic viscoelastic device (OVD) can protect the endothelium cells during the procedure. It also can flat the anterior capsule to make capsulorhexis more controlled. The OVD should be removed completely when surgery finished to prevent intraocular pressure from increasing. If the toric multifocal IOLs used, the OVD should be totally removed behind lens to avoid the accident rotation after surgery [67].

8. Management of dissatisfied patients

Even with fully preoperative examination, careful patient's selection and precisely uneventful surgery, there are always some unhappy patients with their postoperative outcomes.

The main complaints associated with presbyopia correctiong IOLs include blurred vision, photic phenomenon. Blurred vision may be present at near, intermediate, and far distances, or specific distance. It was attributed to refractive error or residual astigmatism, posterior capsule opacification, dry eye, or coexisting ocular disease. It was also caused by loss of contrast sensitivity.

The premium IOLs very affected by small residual ametropias. Surgeon must carefully calculate IOL power by using advanced biometry formulas, customize constant according to previous experience. Any astigmatism greater than 0.75 D in a blur vision patient should be treated. The most common intervention to management of residual refractive error is spectacles or contact lens. Bioptics refractive enhancement can be performed in spherical or cylinder error patients, while IOL exchange or piggyback solution also can be used in case of important defect or if the previous solutions are not possible [17].

Another common cause of blur vision after multifocal lens implantation is ocular surface disease. The symptos can be resolved by treating with lubricating artificial tears, punctal plugs, warm compress and vectored thermal pulsation treatments.

Patients with multifocal IOLs appear more sensitive to posterior capsule opacity than with monofocal IOLs. If posterior capsule opacification is suspected to be the cause of visual disturbance, and symptoms have been worsening since surgery, the surgeon should consider Nd:YAG laser capsulotomy. If there is any chance that a lens exchange may be done, YAG capsulotomy should be delayed, as an open posterior capsule makes the exchange more difficult.

Photic phenomena can consist of glare, halos, and dysphotopsias. It also caused by IOL decentration, dry eye, posterior capsule opacification, or multifocal IOL design. During the procedure, carefully management should be taken including capsule tension ring implantation, centration of the IOLs relative to the visual axis, polishing the anterior and posterior capsule. Most case of photic phenomena will be tolerance or disappear by the time. After the reason of dry eye and PCO had be excluded, the night-time dysphotopsia and decreasing of contrast sensitivity are due to intrinsic properties of multifocal IOL. The most effective aid in managing these problems is neuroadaptation which is highly dependent on the individual and often need time to adapt. If a patient is still bothered by these problems more than three months after surgery, or if their quality of life is significantly affected, an IOL exchange for a monofocal IOL is almost always an alternative [50].

Proper management of the unhappy premium IOL patient requires time, patience, and familiarity with different medical and surgical options and techniques. The most important things are extensive preoperative patient education and avoiding the inadequate patient. Careful patient selection and clear communication regarding realistic expectations are the keys to success with premium IOLs.

9. Summary

Premium multifocal IOLs are a popular option for cataract or presbyopia patients today. Patients can achieve high levels of success and satisfaction from these IOLs. However, adequate preoperative clinical evaluation including patient selection, optical and anatomical examination is crucial to reach a success case. Based on the preoperative diagnosis including the corneal astigmatism, biometry measurement, IOL power calculation, presbyopia correcting IOLs' indications and contraindications should be assessment for IOL selection strategy. Surgical procedure should be technically optimized to achieve the best outcomes. Adequate management of both satisfied and unsatisfied patients will improve the benefit of current premium IOLs.

Author details

Chen Xu[1,2]

1 Aier School of Ophthalmology, Central South University, Changsha, China

2 Department of Opthalmology, Shanghai Aier Eye Hospital, Shanghai, China

*Address all correspondence to: francois.chenxu@gmail.com

References

[1] Jorge LA, Auffarth GU, Bellucci R. State of the Premium IOL Market in Europe 2013. Available from: https://crstodayeurope.com/articles/2013-jan/state-of-the-premium-iol-market-in-europe/.

[2] Wang SY, Stem MS, Oren G, Shtein R, Lichter PR. Patient-centered and visual quality outcomes of premium cataract surgery: a systematic review. Eur J Ophthalmol. 2017;27(4):387-401.

[3] Lawless M, Levitz L, Hodge C. Reviewing the visual benefits of femtosecond laser-assisted cataract surgery: Can we improve our outcomes? Indian J Ophthalmol. 2017;65(12):1314-22.

[4] Shetty N, Kaweri L, Koshy A, Shetty R, Nuijts R, Roy AS. Repeatability of biometry measured by IOLMaster 700, Lenstar LS 900 and Anterion, and its impact on predicted intraocular lens power. J Cataract Refract Surg. 2020.

[5] Alio J, Pikkel J. Multifocal Intraocular Lenses: The Art and Practice. 1 ed. Alio J, Pikkel J, editors. Switzerland: Springer International Publishing; 2014.

[6] Pepose JS, Burke J, Qazi M. Accommodating Intraocular Lenses. Asia Pac J Ophthalmol (Phila). 2017;6(4):350-7.

[7] Pallikaris IG, Kontadakis GA, Portaliou DM. Real and pseudoaccommodation in accommodative lenses. J Ophthalmol. 2011;2011:284961.

[8] Alio JL, Plaza-Puche AB, Montalban R, Ortega P. Near visual outcomes with single-optic and dual-optic accommodating intraocular lenses. J Cataract Refract Surg. 2012;38(9):1568-75.

[9] de Wit DW, Diaz J, Moore TC, Moutari S, Moore JE. Effect of position of near addition in an asymmetric refractive multifocal intraocular lens on quality of vision. J Cataract Refract Surg. 2015;41(5):945-55.

[10] Breyer DRH, Kaymak H, Ax T, Kretz FTA, Auffarth GU, Hagen PR. Multifocal Intraocular Lenses and Extended Depth of Focus Intraocular Lenses. Asia Pac J Ophthalmol (Phila). 2017;6(4):339-49.

[11] Kanclerz P, Toto F, Grzybowski A, Alio JL. Extended Depth-of-Field Intraocular Lenses: An Update. Asia Pac J Ophthalmol (Phila). 2020;9(3):194-202.

[12] MacRae S, Holladay JT, Glasser A, Calogero D, Hilmantel G, Masket S, et al. Special Report: American Academy of Ophthalmology Task Force Consensus Statement for Extended Depth of Focus Intraocular Lenses. Ophthalmology. 2017;124(1):139-41.

[13] Bohm M, Petermann K, Hemkeppler E, Kohnen T. Defocus curves of 4 presbyopia-correcting IOL designs: Diffractive panfocal, diffractive trifocal, segmental refractive, and extended-depth-of-focus. J Cataract Refract Surg. 2019;45(11):1625-36.

[14] Alio JL. Presbyopic Lenses: Evidence, Masquerade News, and Fake News. Asia Pac J Ophthalmol (Phila). 2019;8(4):273-4.

[15] Zvornicanin J, Zvornicanin E. Premium intraocular lenses: The past, present and future. J Curr Ophthalmol. 2018;30(4):287-96.

[16] Yeu E, Cuozzo S. Matching the Patient to the Intraocular Lens: Preoperative Considerations to Optimize Surgical Outcomes. Ophthalmology. 2020.

[17] Braga-Mele R, Chang D, Dewey S, Foster G, Henderson BA, Hill W, et al. Multifocal intraocular lenses: relative indications and contraindications for implantation. J Cataract Refract Surg. 2014;40(2):313-22.

[18] Rychwalski PJ. Multifocal IOL implantation in children: is the future clear? J Cataract Refract Surg. 2010;36(12):2019-21.

[19] Hunter DG. Multifocal intraocular lenses in children. Ophthalmology. 2001;108(8):1373-4.

[20] Jacobi PC, Dietlein TS, Konen W. Multifocal intraocular lens implantation in pediatric cataract surgery. Ophthalmology. 2001;108(8):1375-80.

[21] Cristobal JA, Remon L, Del Buey MA, Montes-Mico R. Multifocal intraocular lenses for unilateral cataract in children. J Cataract Refract Surg. 2010;36(12):2035-40.

[22] Cummings AB. Lifestyle Match Index: Helping to Choose the Best IOL. CATARACT & REFRACTIVE SURGERY TODAY. 2020:44-5,73.

[23] de Vries NE, Webers CA, Touwslager WR, Bauer NJ, de Brabander J, Berendschot TT, et al. Dissatisfaction after implantation of multifocal intraocular lenses. J Cataract Refract Surg. 2011;37(5):859-65.

[24] Holladay JT, Moran JR, Kezirian GM. Analysis of aggregate surgically induced refractive change, prediction error, and intraocular astigmatism. J Cataract Refract Surg. 2001;27(1):61-79.

[25] Roberts HW, Wagh VK, Sullivan DL, Archer TJ, O'Brart DPS. Refractive outcomes after limbal relaxing incisions or femtosecond laser arcuate keratotomy to manage corneal astigmatism at the time of cataract surgery. J Cataract Refract Surg. 2018;44(8):955-63.

[26] Holland E, Lane S, Horn JD, Ernest P, Arleo R, Miller KM. The AcrySof Toric intraocular lens in subjects with cataracts and corneal astigmatism: a randomized, subject-masked, parallel-group, 1-year study. Ophthalmology. 2010;117(11):2104-11.

[27] Crema AS, Walsh A, Ventura BV, Santhiago MR. Visual outcomes of eyes implanted with a toric multifocal intraocular lens. J Refract Surg. 2014;30(7):486-91.

[28] Garzon N, Arriola-Villalobos P, Felipe G, Poyales F, Garcia-Montero M. Intraocular lens power calculation in eyes with keratoconus. J Cataract Refract Surg. 2020;46(5):778-83.

[29] Hashemi H, Heidarian S, Seyedian MA, Yekta A, Khabazkhoob M. Evaluation of the Results of Using Toric IOL in the Cataract Surgery of Keratoconus Patients. Eye Contact Lens. 2015;41(6):354-8.

[30] He C, Joergensen JS, Knorz MC, McKay KN, Zhang F. Three-Step Treatment of Keratoconus and Post-LASIK Ectasia: Implantation of ICRS, Corneal Cross-linking, and Implantation of Toric Posterior Chamber Phakic IOLs. J Refract Surg. 2020;36(2):104-9.

[31] Holladay JT, Dudeja DR, Chang J. Functional vision and corneal changes after laser in situ keratomileusis determined by contrast sensitivity, glare testing, and corneal topography. J Cataract Refract Surg. 1999;25(5):663-9.

[32] Vrijman V, van der Linden JW, van der Meulen IJE, Mourits MP, Lapid-Gortzak R. Multifocal intraocular lens implantation after previous corneal refractive laser surgery for myopia. J Cataract Refract Surg. 2017;43(7):909-14.

[33] Baartman BJ, Karpuk K, Eichhorn B, Ferguson TJ, Sudhagoni RG, Berdahl JP,

et al. Extended depth of focus lens implantation after radial keratotomy. Clin Ophthalmol. 2019;13:1401-8.

[34] Palomino-Bautista C, Carmona-Gonzalez D, Sanchez-Jean R, Castillo-Gomez A, Romero-Dominguez M, Elias de Tejada M, et al. Refractive predictability and visual outcomes of an extended range of vision intraocular lens in eyes with previous myopic laser in situ keratomileusis. Eur J Ophthalmol. 2019;29(6):593-9.

[35] Son HS, Khoramnia R, Mayer C, Labuz G, Yildirim TM, Auffarth GU. A pinhole implant to correct postoperative residual refractive error in an RK cataract patient. Am J Ophthalmol Case Rep. 2020;20:100890.

[36] Starr CE, Gupta PK, Farid M, Beckman KA, Chan CC, Yeu E, et al. An algorithm for the preoperative diagnosis and treatment of ocular surface disorders. J Cataract Refract Surg. 2019;45(5):669-84.

[37] Milner MS, Beckman KA, Luchs JI, Allen QB, Awdeh RM, Berdahl J, et al. Dysfunctional tear syndrome: dry eye disease and associated tear film disorders - new strategies for diagnosis and treatment. Curr Opin Ophthalmol. 2017;27 Suppl 1:3-47.

[38] Fernandez J, Rodriguez-Vallejo M, Martinez J, Burguera N, Pinero DP. Pupil dependence assessment with multifocal intraocular lenses through visual acuity and contrast sensitivity defocus curves. Eur J Ophthalmol. 2020:1120672120940202.

[39] Pazo EE, McNeely RN, Richoz O, Nesbit MA, Moore TCB, Moore JE. Pupil influence on the quality of vision in rotationally asymmetric multifocal IOLs with surface-embedded near segment. J Cataract Refract Surg. 2017;43(11):1420-9.

[40] Qi Y, Lin J, Leng L, Zhao G, Wang Q, Li C, et al. Role of angle kappa in visual quality in patients with a trifocal diffractive intraocular lens. J Cataract Refract Surg. 2018;44(8):949-54.

[41] Fu Y, Kou J, Chen D, Wang D, Zhao Y, Hu M, et al. Influence of angle kappa and angle alpha on visual quality after implantation of multifocal intraocular lenses. J Cataract Refract Surg. 2019;45(9):1258-64.

[42] Prakash G, Prakash DR, Agarwal A, Kumar DA, Agarwal A, Jacob S. Predictive factor and kappa angle analysis for visual satisfactions in patients with multifocal IOL implantation. Eye (Lond). 2011;25(9):1187-93.

[43] Prakash G, Agarwal A, Prakash DR, Kumar DA, Agarwal A, Jacob S. Role of angle kappa in patient dissatisfaction with refractive-design multifocal intraocular lenses. J Cataract Refract Surg. 2011;37(9):1739-40; author reply 40.

[44] Garzon N, Garcia-Montero M, Lopez-Artero E, Albarran-Diego C, Perez-Cambrodi R, Illarramendi I, et al. Influence of angle kappa on visual and refractive outcomes after implantation of a diffractive trifocal intraocular lens. J Cataract Refract Surg. 2020;46(5):721-7.

[45] Wang R, Long T, Gu X, Ma T. Changes in angle kappa and angle alpha before and after cataract surgery. J Cataract Refract Surg. 2020;46(3):365-71.

[46] Grzybowski A, Eppig T. Angle alpha as predictor for improving patient satisfaction with multifocal intraocular lenses? Graefes Arch Clin Exp Ophthalmol. 2021.

[47] Piracha AR. Using angle alpha in premium IOL screening. Cataract and Refractive Surgery Today. 2016:24-5.

[48] Dyrda A, Martinez-Palmer A, Martin-Moral D, Rey A, Morilla A, Castilla-Marti M, et al. Clinical Results of Diffractive, Refractive, Hybrid Multifocal, and Monofocal Intraocular Lenses. J Ophthalmol. 2018;2018:8285637.

[49] Ichhpujani P, Bhartiya S, Sharma A. Premium IOLs in Glaucoma. J Curr Glaucoma Pract. 2013;7(2):54-7.

[50] Alio JL, Plaza-Puche AB, Fernandez-Buenaga R, Pikkel J, Maldonado M. Multifocal intraocular lenses: An overview. Surv Ophthalmol. 2017;62(5):611-34.

[51] Hardin JS, Gauldin DW, Soliman MK, Chu CJ, Yang YC, Sallam AB. Cataract Surgery Outcomes in Eyes With Primary Epiretinal Membrane. JAMA Ophthalmol. 2018;136(2):148-54.

[52] Olsen T. Calculation of intraocular lens power: a review. Acta Ophthalmol Scand. 2007;85(5):472-85.

[53] Chen YA, Hirnschall N, Findl O. Evaluation of 2 new optical biometry devices and comparison with the current gold standard biometer. J Cataract Refract Surg. 2011;37(3):513-7.

[54] Jasvinder S, Khang TF, Sarinder KK, Loo VP, Subrayan V. Agreement analysis of LENSTAR with other techniques of biometry. Eye (Lond). 2011;25(6):717-24.

[55] Kunert KS, Peter M, Blum M, Haigis W, Sekundo W, Schutze J, et al. Repeatability and agreement in optical biometry of a new swept-source optical coherence tomography-based biometer versus partial coherence interferometry and optical low-coherence reflectometry. J Cataract Refract Surg. 2016;42(1):76-83.

[56] Carmona-Gonzalez D, Castillo-Gomez A, Palomino-Bautista C, Romero-Dominguez M, Gutierrez-Moreno MA. Comparison of the accuracy of 11 intraocular lens power calculation formulas. Eur J Ophthalmol. 2020:1120672120962030.

[57] Melles RB, Holladay JT, Chang WJ. Accuracy of Intraocular Lens Calculation Formulas. Ophthalmology. 2018;125(2):169-78.

[58] Savini G, Hoffer KJ. Intraocular lens power calculation in eyes with previous corneal refractive surgery. Eye Vis (Lond). 2018;5:18.

[59] Tang M, Wang L, Koch DD, Li Y, Huang D. Intraocular lens power calculation after previous myopic laser vision correction based on corneal power measured by Fourier-domain optical coherence tomography. J Cataract Refract Surg. 2012;38(4):589-94.

[60] Wang XZ, Cui R, Song XD, Yun B, Qian J, Ding N. Comparison of the accuracy of intraocular lens power calculation formulas for eyes after corneal refractive surgery. Ann Transl Med. 2020;8(14):871.

[61] Savini G, Taroni L, Hoffer KJ. Recent developments in intraocular lens power calculation methods-update 2020. Ann Transl Med. 2020;8(22):1553.

[62] Mahrous A, Ciralsky JB, Lai EC. Revisiting monovision for presbyopia. Curr Opin Ophthalmol. 2018;29(4):313-7.

[63] Smith CE, Allison RS, Wilkinson F, Wilcox LM. Monovision: Consequences for depth perception from large disparities. Exp Eye Res. 2019;183:62-7.

[64] Burge J, Rodriguez-Lopez V, Dorronsoro C. Monovision and the Misperception of Motion. Curr Biol. 2019;29(15):2586-92 e4.

[65] Freitas GO, Boteon JE, Carvalho MJ, Pinto RM. Treatment of astigmatism

during phacoemulsification. Arq Bras Oftalmol. 2014;77(1):40-6.

[66] Gangwani V, Hirnschall N, Findl O, Maurino V. Multifocal toric intraocular lenses versus multifocal intraocular lenses combined with peripheral corneal relaxing incisions to correct moderate astigmatism. J Cataract Refract Surg. 2014;40(10):1625-32.

[67] Visser N, Bauer NJ, Nuijts RM. Toric intraocular lenses: historical overview, patient selection, IOL calculation, surgical techniques, clinical outcomes, and complications. J Cataract Refract Surg. 2013;39(4):624-37.

[68] Li S, Jie Y. Cataract surgery and lens implantation. Curr Opin Ophthalmol. 2019;30(1):39-43.

[69] Lee JA, Song WK, Kim JY, Kim MJ, Tchah H. Femtosecond laser-assisted cataract surgery versus conventional phacoemulsification: Refractive and aberrometric outcomes with a diffractive multifocal intraocular lens. J Cataract Refract Surg. 2019;45(1):21-7.